Discover 5 Essential Concepts
for Torching Body Fat & Keeping it Off
FOREVER
The Mind & Body Connection
Understanding the Female Body
Diet & Nutrition
Exercise
Lifestyle

I0423622

How to be Fit, Fabulous, Fortified, & Free

The Ultimate Women's Guide to Discovering the physical
and spiritual connection to fat loss and a healthy lifestyle

Ericka S. Payne
Certified Personal Trainer, ACSM

Lifestyle Publishing
an imprint of
TLF Limited Management
Edgewood, Maryland

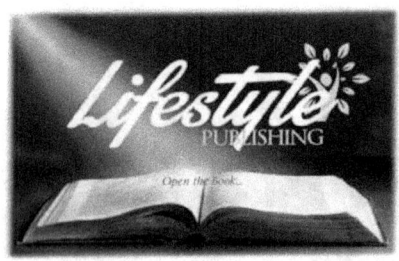

A subsidiary of TLF Limited Management
1913 Hawthorne Road
Edgewood MD 21040

First edition paperback June 2017

LIFESTYLE PUBLISHING
For information on special discounts for bulk purchases, please contact TLF Limited Management, reference Lifestyle Publishing, tlflimited@gmail.com.

Designed by Tracy L.F. Worley

Manufactured in the United States of America

Library of Congress Case Number: 1-5330325131

ISBN-978-1547195831

Testimonials

"Ericka is great!!! I am enjoying group classes with Ericka! She is very inspiring and encourages you to work your hardest. Not the person next to you or behind you, but your personal best! She stresses the importance of technique. I really enjoy my classes with Ericka. I have definitely found that with Payne there is gain and loss, both in a good way!" ~ Debbie C.

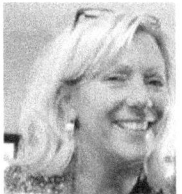

"My experience with Ericka has been nothing but positive. Ericka has taken me to new levels that I would never have imagined possible. She encourages me to give 100% but continues to be positive and motivational even when I feel like giving up." ~ Terri P.

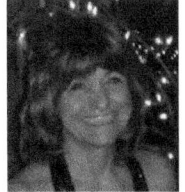

"I think you are the greatest! I feel like I'm getting stronger in my wonderful old age, thanks to your class." ~ Annette

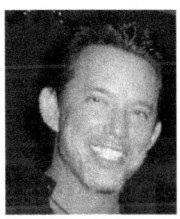

"Ericka is very in tune to the individual needs of her class. Although each person in her class may have separate goals, she personally instructs and suggests changes in training to each member of her class based on their individual goals." ~ Joe L.

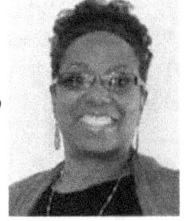

"My health and wellness journey with Ericka has been life changing. She has been instrumental in helping me to achieve my fitness goals. I'm inspired by the level of commitment and passion she has for helping people. If you do what she tells you to do, you WILL get the desired results! You will be a healthier, happier you! Ericka understands that one size does not fit all. After your initial consultation and comprehensive assessment she will develop a personalized, customized fitness program to help you achieve your fitness goals. This has become a lifestyle for me. I'm 52 years old and blessed to be in the best health of my life! Life is so precious, and each day is a gift from God. Take care of your temple and it will take care of you!" ~ Michele!!

More Testimonials

"Ericka is a professional, tough, no nonsense thorough trainer who will push you hard to get results. She works to help you arrive at what works for you. If one is serious, Ericka is worth it because of the results. She educates you and helps you see and learn what your needs are. It is a long and tough road but she can and has helped me to make the lifestyle change to be successful." ~ Nick S.

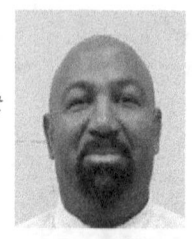

"I'm learning so much from her and love training with her. She has a wealth of information on fitness and nutrition that is going to really help me reach my goals!!" ~ Debbie S.

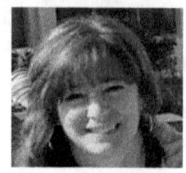

"We absolutely love working with you. You are the good kind of Payne!!" ~ Joe & Ica

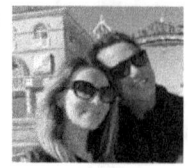

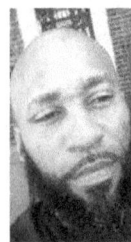

"I lost 18 pounds working with Ericka!" ~ William H.

"Ericka was honest from the moment I walked into her office and was eager to meet my goals. In other words, she will walk beside you and run with you when she knew you were capable of taking the next step. If you need someone truthful and faithful til the end, she is that person." ~ Denise W.

2017 Couple's FAT LOSS SUCCESS STORY

I wanted to congratulate two of Figure 8 Fizique's Superstars who've lost a total of 92 pounds!!! Simply Phenomenal! This husband and wife team have smashed all expectations and they are still dropping weight. Michele has lost over 52 pounds and 10 inches on her journey. Ladies, this true n' real classy lady warrior is committed, determined, and intent on reaching her goals and she is doing it! She has totally embraced being proactive about her physical and spiritual well being, and it emanates!! Nick (diagnosed with hypothyroidism) has lost a total of 37 pounds and over 10 inches *naturally*! He does not take any synthetic medication at all! How you like that?!?! Nick uses a holistic approach to his health and wellness and though he has to work harder than most, he's committed and gets results. The man is relentless, dead set on his goals, and focused on conquering his weight loss!!! Kudos Nick!! By the way, folks, they're both in their 50s!! Congratulations again, Nick and Michele!! ~ *Ericka*

About the Author

My name is Ericka Payne and I'm going to be radically honest with you.

For 12 years I struggled with my weight and self image, and pretty much gave up trying and let myself go. Then it happened. I caught myself constantly not wanting to look in the mirror. I was horrified when I saw myself, and ashamed to see how out of control my health had gotten. Over the next several months I spiraled even further, becoming more and more depressed about my weight. The more I looked in the mirror, the more I ate. I just accepted my body. I would be fat for the rest of my life.

But then a friend recommended a trainer she came across. I figured, what else do I have to lose? I signed up and the rest is history! My trainer, now good friend, patiently blasted over 65 pounds off my body with effective fat torching formulas.

Today, I continue my fitness journey as a personal trainer and humble student learning cutting edge fat loss formulas that work. You've seen countless before and after photos of me and there are more powerful testimonies to come from others now torching body fat using my fat loss formula. So, what's the formula?
1. No More Diets, They don't work.
2. No More hours on the treadmill 5 to 7 days a week. It makes you fat.
3. No More B12 shots, wraps, surgeries, etc. All are quick fixes to a long-standing issues between your two ears.

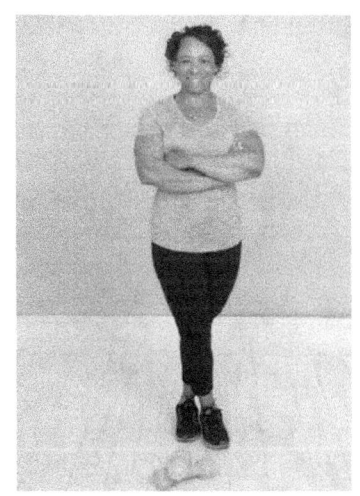

Simply put, I have identified and proven the best resistance, intensity interval cardio, and nutrition plans that save time, burn fat, tone muscle, flatten your belly, and balance your hormonal system to keep a healthy, lean, toned body that feeds the muscle and starves the fat. The biggest challenge for many people is the matter located between your two ears. When you learn how to master the helm and become the captain of your ship, you'll begin to make good, better, and best choices, and commit to your fat loss journey. I will show you in this book how to conquer your weight loss fears and become *Fit, Fabulous, Fortified and Free!*

Let's get started!

Ericka

DEDICATION

"For I know the thoughts that I think toward you, saith the LORD, thoughts of peace, and not of evil, to give you an expected end. Then shall ye call upon me, and ye shall go and pray unto me, and I will hearken unto you. And ye shall seek me, and find me, when ye shall search for me with all your heart. And I will be found of you, saith the LORD…" -JEREMIAH 29:11-14

To the One and Only God Almighty of the heavens and earth….I am nonexistent without you. Thank you for sending your son The Lord and Savior Jesus the Christ who paved the way for salvation. Thank you Lord God for your grace and mercy. Thank you Lord God for deliverance from sin, destruction and damnation. Thank you Lord God for eternal life found only in your son Jesus. Thank you Lord God for One Lord, One Faith, One Baptism, The One Way, The One Truth, The One Life, The One Door to heaven Jesus, The Christ. Thank You Lord God for the road map, the standard, the undisputable word of God. If a man and woman will hear, believe and put on the Holy Spirit in baptism thus he/she will unlock all the doors once closed and began a beautiful journey to glory. Thank you Lord God for the church of Christ where life begins and never ends. My life is forever indebted to you body, soul and spirit until the last amen.

To my mom, Leiola J. Mathews, my sole champion and giver in my corner always pushing me, encouraging me, picking me up when I'm down, putting a little wood in the fire to keep it burning till I'm flaming again. I am forever grateful and thankful to have you as my Mom. I love you so much! Thank you for instilling the tenacity go-getter attitude and relentlessness in your daughter to fight on! This one's for you!

To my personal trainer and good friend, Ed Robinson of Charm City Women's Fitness, this one's for you! Thank you for believing in me, sticking with me, and pushing me even when I'd given up long ago. You have a gift of helping people reach their fitness goals, and you are a living inspiration to many in making it a lifestyle. You inspired me, and I sincerely thank you. To my true and real dear friends which are many, I can write a book alone on so many men and women who've been a rock and foundation in my life building me to the woman I am to-day. For what ever reason, season or a life time you have traveled with me on my journey, I personally thank you. This book and all its splendor could not have been written without going through many trials, tribulations, lessons learned, winning some, losing some, but never giving up, life experiences good or bad yet holding on to the true and real relationships I had in you. Again, thank you. This book is dedicated to you.

CONTENTS

Mind, Body & Soul Interconnection

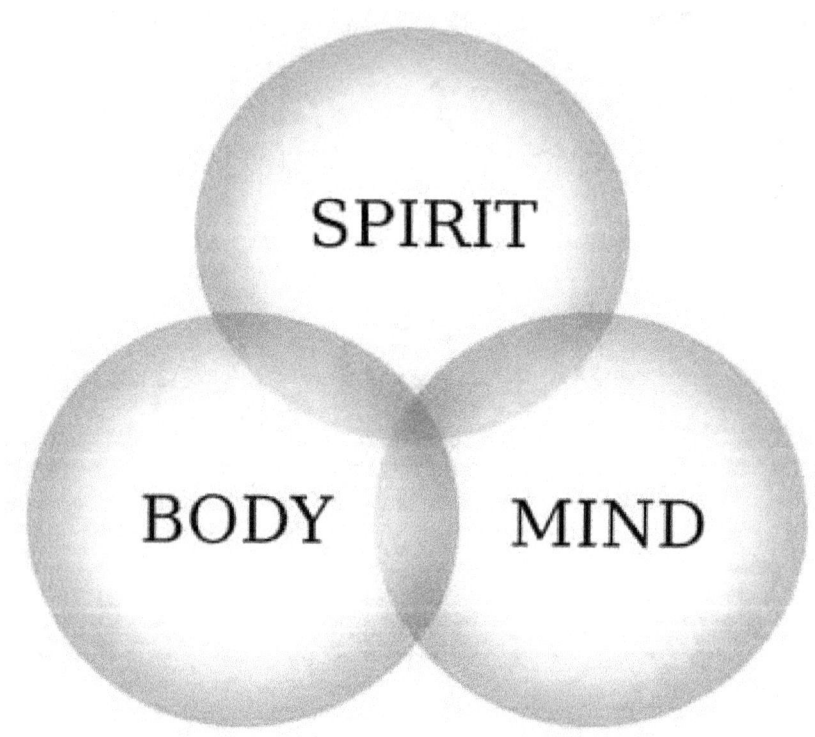

(1)

What does the mind have to do with fat loss?

"And God said, Let us make man in our image, after our likeness: and let them have dominion over the fish of the sea, and over the fowl of the air, and over the cattle, and over all the earth, and over every creeping thing that creepeth upon the earth. So God created man in his own image, in the image of God created he him; male and female created he them (God's spiritual image). And the LORD God formed man of the dust of the ground, and breathed into his nostrils the breath of life; and man became a living soul" (Genesis 1:26-27; 2:7).

Before you began to deal with anything you need some information first. Good place to start is with Who, What, When, Where, Why and How. When God created man he made him a trifold being: body, soul and spirit. All three are connected and work interchangeably for man to survive and live on this earth. Man is a trichotomy:

Spirit-Pneuma
air, breeze, to blow, life

Soul-Psuche
the soul-the immortal soul; the rational seat of man; the spiritual nature

Body-Soma/Somatikos
physical body

The Physical & Spiritual Connection

In Ecclesiastes 12:1-7 the bible tells us the body is born to die -- the physical body or vessel was not designed to last forever and as life goes on man's body/vessel is slowly bending toward the grave. *"The days of our years are threescore years and ten; and if by reason of strength they be fourscore years, yet is their strength labour and sorrow; for it is soon cut off, and we fly away"* (Psalm 90:10). At best, if an individual lives to see 70-80 years old, he/she has lived out their life expectancy. Now we know there are some instances where people are living well in their early 100's. That is a rare blessing. It seems they've done some good things taking care of their bodies in order to achieve such longevity.

What about the millions dying well under life expectancy because of modifiable behaviors that cause health risks, such as tobacco use, obesity, inactivity, high blood pressure, diabetes, high cholesterol, chronic stress? We'll revisit this topic in a later chapter.

We need our physical bodies to traverse through this lifetime, connect with people, places and things. The physical body is "matter," just as the earth, our dwelling place, is what God called it to be, and man will have dominion over the earth and rule it. Most importantly, the body was designed to worship and serve the one creator of the heavens and the earth, the Lord God Almighty. *"What? Know ye not that your body is the temple of the Holy Ghost which is in you, which ye have of God, and ye are not your own? For ye are bought with a price: therefore glorify God in your body, and in your spirit, which are God's"* (1 Corinthians 6:19-20).

Yes, God has an expectation for man to worship Him in body and spirit. We have a responsibility and accountability to do what He commands. When the Bible says, "glorify in body and spirit," that means to be full of glory, honour, praise, magnify, worship, and dignity. In other words, take care of your body and represent your Creator with your best. However, it does not mean you have to be the fittest of fit, in impeccable shape, and wear a size 6! Simply do your best to be fit and able to do God's will. You can't march in God's army if your weight or physical condition won't allow it.

The apostle Paul sent words of encouragement to the saints at Thessalonica, *"And the very God of peace sanctify you wholly; and I pray God your whole spirit and soul and body be preserved blameless unto the coming of our Lord Jesus Christ"* (1 Thessalonians 5:13). We should strive to be healthy -- the best body, soul, and spirit we can be! *"Beloved, I wish above all things that thou mayest prosper and be in health, even as thy soul prospereth."* The word health or "hygiaínō" in greek means to have sound health; be well in body; figuratively, to be uncorrupt true in doctrine; be safe and sound, be wholesome. Your body is important too, and God wants us to know that. The saints also recognized this and sent encouraging words from time to time to each other.

The most important point I want to make in this book is that God ultimately wants your soul. See, it's not about the physical body at all, though we need it here on earth (1Timothy 4:8), but God tells us there is a part of you that will live beyond the grave, the soul. The choices you make while you still have breath in your body will determine your eternal home. In other words, chasing a figure-eight body with a flat belly and toned hips, butt, and thighs without God at the helm is like chasing the wind only to fall off a cliff to your death. *"Then shall the dust return to the earth as it was: and the spirit shall return unto God who gave it. Let us hear the conclusion of the whole matter: Fear God, and keep his commandments: for this is the whole duty of man. For God shall bring every work into judgment, with every secret thing, whether it be good, or whether it be evil"* (Ecclesiastes 12:7; 13-14). *"And as it is appointed unto men once to die, but after this the judgment"* (Hebrews 9:27).

What Does God Expect from Me?

The Sin Problem

Mankind has a sin problem that separates us from the love of God and eternal life (Romans 3:10, 23; Romans 6:23). When Adam and Eve disobeyed God in the Garden of Eden and ate of the tree of the knowledge of good and evil, sin passed to all mankind and separated us from God. All praises, honor and glory be to God for His grace and mercy, because He already had a plan to get His best creation back into relationship with Him. The plan of salvation was given to all men and women in His Son, Jesus. *"Neither is there salvation in any other: for there is none other name under heaven given among men, whereby we must be saved"* (Acts 4:12).

The Authority

Who has the power and authority to orchestrate my life? To whom will I give this power to and why should I listen to him?

Hear Him
"While he yet spake, behold, a bright cloud overshadowed them: and behold a voice out of the cloud, which said, This is my beloved Son, in whom I am well pleased; hear ye him." (Mark 9:7)

All Power
"And Jesus came and spake unto them, saying, All power is given unto me in heaven and in earth." (Matthew 28:18)

The Door
"I am the door: by me if any man enter in, he shall be saved, and shall go in and out, and find pasture." (John 10:9)

One Way
"...I am the way, the truth, and the life: no man cometh unto the Father, but by me." (John 14:6)

The Divine Solution

Jesus, the Son of God, is the answer to all our hopes, desires, dreams, passions, trials, and tribulation, and ultimately our love affair with Him leads to eternal life. If you never obey the gospel of Jesus, the Christ, you'll never have a chance to reach your physical and spiritual potential and will forever be separated, lost, and condemned in a sinful state, damned to eternal damnation.

As I mentioned before, it's not about the physical, for the body is a means to an end. Yes, you can have a fit, tone, lean figure and be in fantastic shape, ready for the world. But none of that will matter outside the Body of Christ. Your soul salvation matters far more than the physical. *"Repent, and be baptized every one of you in the name of Jesus Christ for the remission of sins, and ye shall receive the gift of the Holy Ghost…..Save yourselves from this untoward generation"* (Acts 2:28, 40). The most important decision you'll ever make in your life is to obey the word of God, the gospel of Jesus, the Christ. Humble yourself to him, learn of him, get to know him, his will and plan for you. Upon your obedience to his words, he promised to give you the Holy Spirit to guide your footsteps and help you live as He commands. He will love you, encourage you, teach you, protect you, and guide you until he calls you home.

What is God's Plan of Salvation?

Hear the Word of God
Romans 10:17
John 6:44-45
Acts 2:37-47

Believe the Word of God
Mark 16:16
Hebrews 11:6
James 2:14-26

Repent/Change your Life
Acts 2:38
Luke 13:3
Acts 3:19

Confess that Jesus is the Son of God
Acts 8:37
Romans 10:10
Luke 22:8-9

Be Baptized in the Body of Christ for the Remission of Sins
1 Peter 3:20-21
Matthew 28:18-20
Galatians 3:27

Live Faithfully for the rest of your Life
Rev 2:10
Hebrews 3:6, 14
2 Timothy 4:6-8

"For God so loved the world that he gave his only begotten Son, that whosoever believeth in him should not perish, but have everlasting life. For God sent not his Son into the world to condemn the world; but that the world through him might be saved. He that believeth on him is not condemned: but he that believeth not is condemned already, because he hath not believed in the name of the only begotten Son of God" (John 3:16-18).

Will you obey? If you want to study and learn more about the Word of God and be obedient to His Word, contact the **Church of Christ** in your community and ask about the one church Jesus promised to build (Matthew 16:18). If you need help locating the Church of Christ in your area please contact me at **Figure 8 Fizique**, figure8fizique4life.com, and we will be happy to point you in the right direction.

Change Your Thinking

When you receive the Holy Spirit, God's seal and stamp of approval, you belong to Him, and you begin to conquer life, self-image and self-esteem issues, fat loss, and anything else you put your mind to do (Ephesians 1:10-14). *"I beseech you therefore, brethren, by the mercies of God, that ye present your bodies a living sacrifice, holy, acceptable unto God, which is your reasonable service. And be not conformed to this world: but be ye transformed by the renewing of your mind, that ye may prove what is that good, and acceptable, and perfect, will of God"* (Romans 12:1).

When you de-program your mind of lies, evil, negative, and dysfunctional thinking, and re-program it with real love, truth, positivity, and good, clean, wholesome thinking, you'll begin to learn and mature to the individual God would have you to be (Philippians 4:8). When you use your ability to make sound decisions, and set your heart on doing the best for God, you will evolve to the essence of your being in all you do, and this thinking will propel your fat loss journey to heights you never thought you could achieve.

What does this have to do with weight loss? If you don't make the spiritual commitment in your mind, carrying out tasks and actions to achieve your goals, you'll never lose the weight and keep it off. You will experience ups and downs, and progress and setbacks that don't work well. The ultimate goal is committing to the journey. Be patient, prepared to learn, and grow with new information from a wide variety of people, places, and things about weight loss, health, and overall wellness. Connect with successful people who have done what you are trying to do, verify their system by listening to and learning from their story, and emulate them when you create your own story.

Yes, copy and paste proven formulas. Live vicariously through your chosen mentor, and be wise, willing to listen to good counsel, and do it. A wise man will take good counsel and put it to use. *"A wise man will hear, and will increase learning; and a man of understanding shall attain unto wise counsels"* (Proverbs 1:15). Don't be a fool only listening but not doing (Proverbs 12:15). Knowledge is not power. It only becomes powerful when you *use it.* Don't be a sponge for information and never do anything with it.

Who is the captain of your ship? Who's at the helm?

Now that you've obeyed the gospel, who's giving the orders? Are you taking orders from the flesh or the Spirit? Before you start your fat loss journey, it's important to understand your role (the Steward), the order taker (the Flesh), and the order giver (the Holy Spirit). Fast foods, fad diets, supplements, and quick fixes will bombard your mind regularly. The biggest challenge you'll have on your fat loss journey is choosing the right people, places, and things to aid you, then filtering what's best.

I heard a gospel preacher some time ago put it this way:
> *"The body is designed to be the slave to the spirit and to take orders from the soul. The soul takes orders from the Spirit which governs, guides, develops and directs the soul. Keep that in the forefront and you'll be a success and help others."*

The Spirit is the Supervisor
The Soul is the Steward
The Body is the Slave

Count the Cost

How badly do you really want to lose the weight? When will it hurt enough for you to take action?

What kinds of investments are you willing to make in yourself? Physically, emotionally, financially?

These are questions and other considerations you really have to make **before** deciding to start your fat loss journey. Why? *"For which of you, intending to build a tower, sitteth not down first, and counteth the cost, whether he have sufficient to finish it? Lest haply, after he hath laid the foundation, and is not able to finish it, all that behold it begin to mock him, Saying, This man began to build, and was not able to finish"* (Luke 14:28-30).

In other words, don't make a mockery of yourself. Sit down, determine what it will cost you, and make the mental and financial commitment. Yes, it's gonna cost you something. Whether you join a gym, get a trainer, or buddy up and explore nature, DO IT! Or else, you are automatically committing to pills, prescribed medicines, endless doctor visits, poor quality of life, physical ailments, and the mental torment of knowing you're not healthy and refusing to do anything about it.

For example, plan it the same way you plan that favorite yearly trip to Las Vegas, Jamaica, or a 10-day cruise to the Caribbean. You methodically outline the details of the trip. You research the cost, sign on to purchase, make the payments, and take the trip. You make a commitment both physically and mentally that you are going on the trip. And you accomplish your goal by doing it. *Is your health less important than a moment in time? Do you care so little about your health that you would rather spend $3500-$5000 on a 2-week vacation and then live the remainder of the year depressed, frustrated, miserable, and disappointed because your health continues to get worse?*

I hope to evolve your thought processes to consider true fitness. And we all know, at the end of the day we do what we want to do. We are willing to pay for anything we believe has value. In some case, we pay for it by any means necessary. Approach your life and take care of your body, soul, and spirit *by any means necessary.* You will set in motion a beautiful journey to becoming **Fit, Fabulous, Fortified, and Free!**

Self -Examination, Positive Self-Talk and Affirmations

Who do you THINK you are? *"As a man thinketh in his heart, so is he"* (Proverbs 23:7).

What are my Values?
Pattern of Beliefs (Belief System) Positive or Negative
What is my Self-Image? How do I see myself?
Why do I think & feel the way I do about my Health? Nutrition, physical activities?
Where is my Faith?

Misbeliefs, Lies, & Falsehoods

"I can't help my weight, it runs in the family."
"I'm just going to be fat, I'll just accept that and live with it."
"I don't have time to go to the gym."
"I can't afford it."
"I can't afford a personal trainer."
"I've tried everything and nothing seems to work."

"Well God will accept me just the way I am."
"I don't have good genes."
"I wish I can have a flat belly and hips like hers."

Changed Thinking, the Power in Positive Self-Talk

"I CAN help my weight regardless of the circumstances."
"With the help of the Holy Spirit, I'm am going to strive to be the best I CAN be in Christ, body, soul, and Spirit."
"I WILL make time to go to the gym & find a way to afford it."
"If education & accountability is what I need, I WILL find the money or resources needed to achieve my goals."
"Although I have some medical limitations, I WILL find the best nutrition and exercise plan best suited for me and do it!"
"I WILL present my body...holy, pleasing, & acceptable to God."
"I thank God for my genetics and I CAN work with them."
"I am fearfully and wonderfully made!"
"I WILL pray always to God to give me the strength and wisdom to accomplish whatever I put my mind to."

I AM, I CAN, I WILL
"I can do all things through Christ who strengthens me" (Philippians 4:13).

No More Excuses

No more "I can't"
No more "I'll get to it when I get to it"
No more "That's not for me because..."
No more "But I..."
No more "I'll try"
No more "I'm broke, no money to start"
No more "When I get a chance
No more "New Year's resolution"
No more "what had happen was"
No more "If only they had"
NO MORE, NO MORE, NO MORE EXCUSES!

What is the secret to weight loss, keeping it off and living up to your God given physical and spiritual potential?
    1) The Mind of Christ is renewed thinking.
    2) Commitment to begin and stay with your weight loss journey.
    3) Lifestyle choices of good nutritional habits, smart exercise, and a healthy balance that works for your body.

Understanding the Female Body & Fat Loss

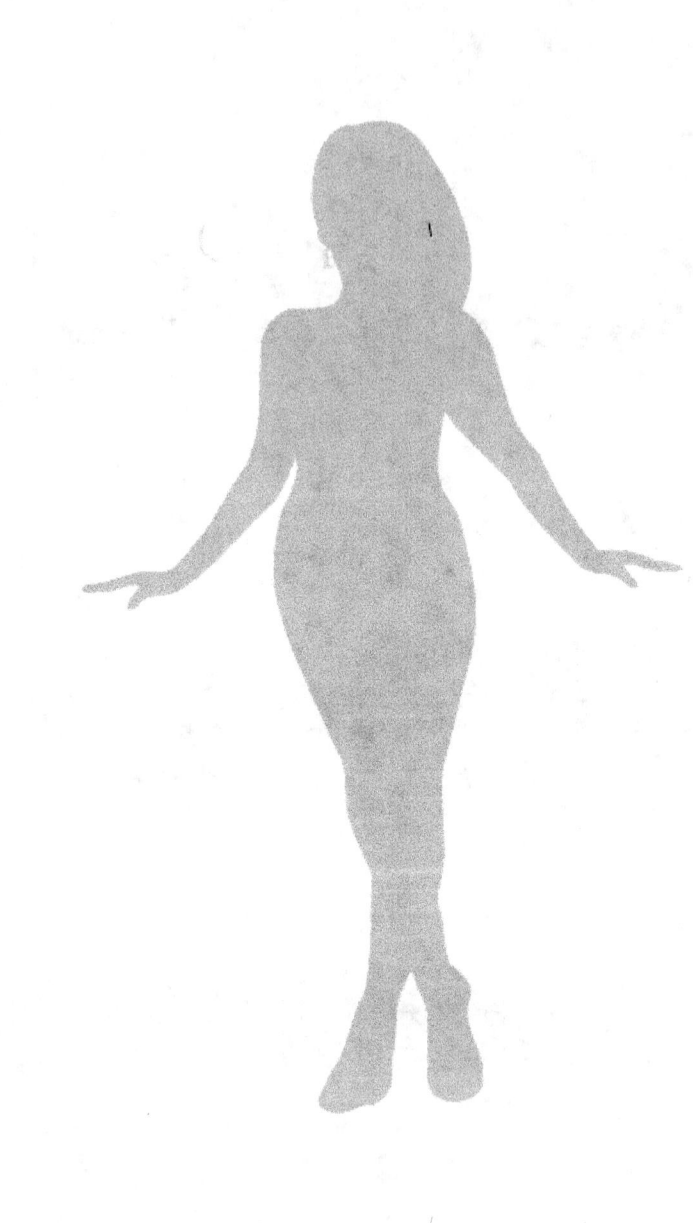

(2)

The woman's body is special, beautiful, and unique, both inside and out. Before you began to choose foods, exercises, and fat loss plans on your weight loss journey, you first need to understand how God created you, how he wired your body and spirit. A woman needs to know how she operates -- genetics, body type, hormones, menstrual cycle, fat and muscle distribution -- and the modifiable and non-modifiable factors that may affect her body throughout life.

The Woman's Hard Wire

"I am fearfully and wonderfully made." (Psalm 139:14).

When Eve took of the fruit in the garden and gave it to her husband, Adam, sin passed to all mankind. Because Adam and Eve disobeyed God's command, *"But of the tree of the knowledge of good and evil, thou shalt not eat of it: for in the day that thou eatest thereof thou shalt surely die"* (Genesis 2:17), God placed the burden on the man to labor and toil all the days of his life until he returns to the grave. To the woman, God greatly multiplied her pain in childbirth and commanded her to submit her desire (will) to her husband.

Unfortunately, the word *submission* has a bad reputation to women because we believe it means we can't think or move without our husband's permission. Not so. God set the order and roles, not because women don't possess the capacity to lead or are spiritually weaker than men, but because Adam was formed first (not Eve) and Eve (not Adam) was deceived by the serpent (1 Timothy 2:8-15). Woman are praised, honored, and recognized in the sight of God when she first lives in reverence to her Creator (Proverbs 31:30). God also considers her to be very special when she lives meekly, quietly, and with in subjection to God first and to her husband (if she's married). It is important to understand this biblical teaching and the role of women, single or married. Accurate interpretation and application of scriptures can unleash the many gift, talents, and abilities a woman may be harboring.

Consider God's love for women: *Woman, you are beautiful because you came from me and I made you that way. I know you can lead in anything you so choose. I made you that way. However, I want you to do something for me, I want you to be obedient to your husband and I want him to lead you as I lead him. I made man and woman. Honor my will for woman and you will be blessed beyond measure.*

Do you realize how great a thing God is asking the woman? Not because she can't say or do anything, but because she can and is more than capable to do anything she sets her heart to do.

The mind of a woman is probably one of the most powerful instruments on this earth. Women have every potential to learn, teach, and lead in their lives, by word and example, the people around her. Women also have the power of influence. Consider the virtuous woman. *"Who can find a virtuous women? For her price is far above rubies"* (Proverbs 31:10). There are so many attributes the Proverbs writer used to describe a *good woman.* The word "virtuous" in this text is defined "chayil" which is Hebrew for force, valor, strength, army, band of soldiers, strong, mighty, worthy, substance, goods, activity, and company of great force. How powerful God has created the potential for a woman!!!

When you read Proverbs 31 you will find a prudent woman, a wife. She is strong physically and spiritually, a wise decision maker, clever yet cautious, skillful in work and business, considerate and attentive to herself, her husband and those around her, a worker bee, not idle; she is prepared, patient, and passionate in everything she does. Her husband is known among men because of her, her children are well reared and cared after. She is a women who fears God and keeps His blessed commands. *Strength and Honor are her clothing...*

You have everything you need to be successful in this life! When you put your God-given mind to a task, you conquer it very well! *Do you understand God's potential for you? Do you see how powerful and influential your example is to the men and women around you? Do you see how you can take your fat loss journey and conquer it?* A woman has everything she needs to be overly successful in all she does -- now, use the tools and become a good woman! Don't let stress, low self-esteem, poor self-image, selling yourself short, idleness, or any external life circumstance take you off track! Put on the whole armor of God! Give the devil no space for trickery (Ephesians 6:10-18; 1 Peter 5:8-10)!!

Genetics

According to Webster's dictionary, genetics is defined as "a branch of biology that deals with the heredity and variation of organisms." We are all created with a code or map from our parents that dictates our body shape/type, and physical characteristics such as skin color, hair, nails, eyes, height, etc. Outside of modern day manipulation with experiments attempting to change and control genetics, you are who you were created to be. You cannot erase who you are. Love, embrace, and accept your womanhood in all its splendor.

Your body doesn't take orders from you to lose weight in specific areas (spot reduction). Fat loss is distributed according to your genetic code and you will lose weight in the areas your body chooses, regardless of what you target profusely with exercise. For example, doing 100 crunches a day will not flatten your belly. The stomach may get harder or even bigger because you are working the abdominal muscle. However, the fat on top of the muscle will still be there. Therefore, let go of the idea, "I just want a flat belly and a butt that sits up." When you begin your fat loss journey and lose weight, those areas can certainly be revealed and developed with the right nutrition and exercise program.

Body Type

According to American psychologist, Williams Sheldon, there are 3 kinds of body types: *endomorph, mesomorph, and ectomorph.*

Endomorphs have a soft, round, stocky build with a fair amount of body fat around their abdomen. Their shape is similar to that of an apple. They have a slow metabolism and tend to gain muscle and fat very easily. They have naturally strong legs. A high protein diet is highly recommend for this body type and workouts should be centered on cardio and weights.

Mesomorphs have strong, muscular, athlete builds with good posture, and broad shoulders. They are fairly symmetric. They are full of energy with thick powerful muscles, evenly distributed throughout their body. They tend to gain muscle easy. They can also become overweight by consuming a high fat diet. This body type responds best to weight training. Their shape is similar to that of an hourglass, the *figure eight* physique.

Ectomorphs are typically skinny, have slight muscles, fragile build, and fast metabolism, and find it hard to gain muscle. They can also lose fat very easily, hence making it difficult to hold on to lean muscle mass. They have to eat at regular intervals, especially before bed to prevent the body from feeding off of muscle for energy. Workouts should be short and intense with an emphasis on building muscle.

Some individuals may carry a mixture of body types such as ectomorph-mesomorph or mesomorph-endomorph. For example, a cross of an ecto-meso may have the ability to gain and retain muscle easily, but have a challenge shredding fat and high water retention.

From these baseline body types, a woman's shape can range anywhere from a stick, oval, pear, rectangle or box shape, to hourglass, or inverted triangle. These shapes are perpetuated by how she's proportioned, her bone structure, build, and overall distribution of body fat. When you discover your body type, it will become more feasible to build a fat loss program with genetics, body type, and current health status conditions, and to stick with your program. We'll discuss diet and exercise in later chapters.

About those Hormones

Hormones play a major part in our total body functionality. According to Webster's Dictionary, hormones are defined as a product of living cells that circulate in body fluids (as blood) and produces a specific often stimulatory effect on the activity of cells usually remote from its point of origin. Without these little messengers communicating almost instantaneously, telling the body what chemicals to release or not to release, we can very easily cease to exist. They are the prime movers in the body for breathing, eating, sleeping, exercising, communicating, awareness, stress, and so many more attributes of daily living. *Hormones are the main catalysts for weight gain or loss.*

There are several brain hormones that play a major role in fat loss. Below is a list of hormones from the National Center for Biotechnology Information (NCBI) that affect weight loss efforts. There are many more key hormones that impact weight loss and work interconnected with each other, therefore this list is not exhaustive.

Insulin
Insulin is produced by the pancreas beta cells; after each meal, insulin is released to help the body store or use energy. It also helps to lower blood sugar levels, and converts glucose and protein to fat which ultimately gets stored away in fat cells or used for energy. Insulin is sometimes referred to as the fat storage hormone because when you eat (especially a diet high in sugars, carbohydrates, and fats), your body races to lower your blood sugar levels by breaking down this energy and storing it away as fat. This hormone works opposite of its counter-hormone, *ghrelin.*

Leptin
Leptin is made in your fat cells and sends messages to your brain to stop eating. It is sometimes referred to as the master hormone because it helps to regulate body weight. When leptin levels are at a certain threshold, the body has enough fat stored and you can use energy at a normal rate, eat regular meals, exercise, etc.

How Insulin & Leptin Resistance Affect Fat Loss
> *When the receptors on cells begin to malfunction or stop responding to insulin, blood sugar will began to rise. If insulin doesn't convert sugar into energy or store as fat, the body will be flooded with excess amounts of sugar. This condition also known as hyperinsulinemia that lead to diabetes, high blood pressure, cholesterol elevation and excessive weight gain. Taking medication for this issue or any other only treats the symptoms not the core issue. The best way to correct this problem is change in diet.* Dr Eades, MD, "Protein Power"

Leptin Resistance

One of the biggest problems overweight and obese individuals have in common is leptin resistance. Overweight people have large amounts of leptin (fat cells) floating around in the body, but the brain is not getting the signal to stop eating. The more weight gained, the higher the leptin levels. We all have a floor, but there is no ceiling for leptin. This means your fat and your brain can't see it. This vicious cycle ultimately leads to obesity. Correcting this problem can be just as daunting because when the body loses fat, you brain still is getting the signal the body is starving, and still hungry with cravings to eat more and exercise less. One of the best ways to balance your leptin levels is to maintain a healthy, balanced diet and exercise program for the long term.

Glucagon

Glucagon works opposite of insulin. It is produced in the part of pancreas known as islets of Langerhans by the alpha cells, and it regulates usage of glucose and fat. When the body detects that blood sugar levels are low, glucagon is released, stimulating the breakdown of glucose, fats, or protein for energy. For fat loss, glucagon can be a catalyst for burning fat because after a period of time following a meal (approximately 2-3 hours when you're not hungry) the body will release this hormone, and burn energy as fuel to keep your metabolism going.

Cortisol

Cortisol is produced by the adrenal glands, and is often referred to as the stress hormone. Cortisol has positive effects such as helping to build muscle and burn fat in the case of exercising for a short or intermediate period of time. For this to be effective, fat loss workouts should stay between 30-45 minutes maximum. Anything beyond this time frame will stress the body. Cortisol will respond to exercise and foods, as well as physical, biological, and mental stress. The negative impact of this hormone is that it releases repetitively in the body. Women who carry excessive weight around the midsection can attribute fat gain and stubborn fat loss to cortisol. Sleep, rest, and a balanced diet with an exercise regimen can help reduce the negative effects of cortisol.

Menstrual Cycle & Hormones

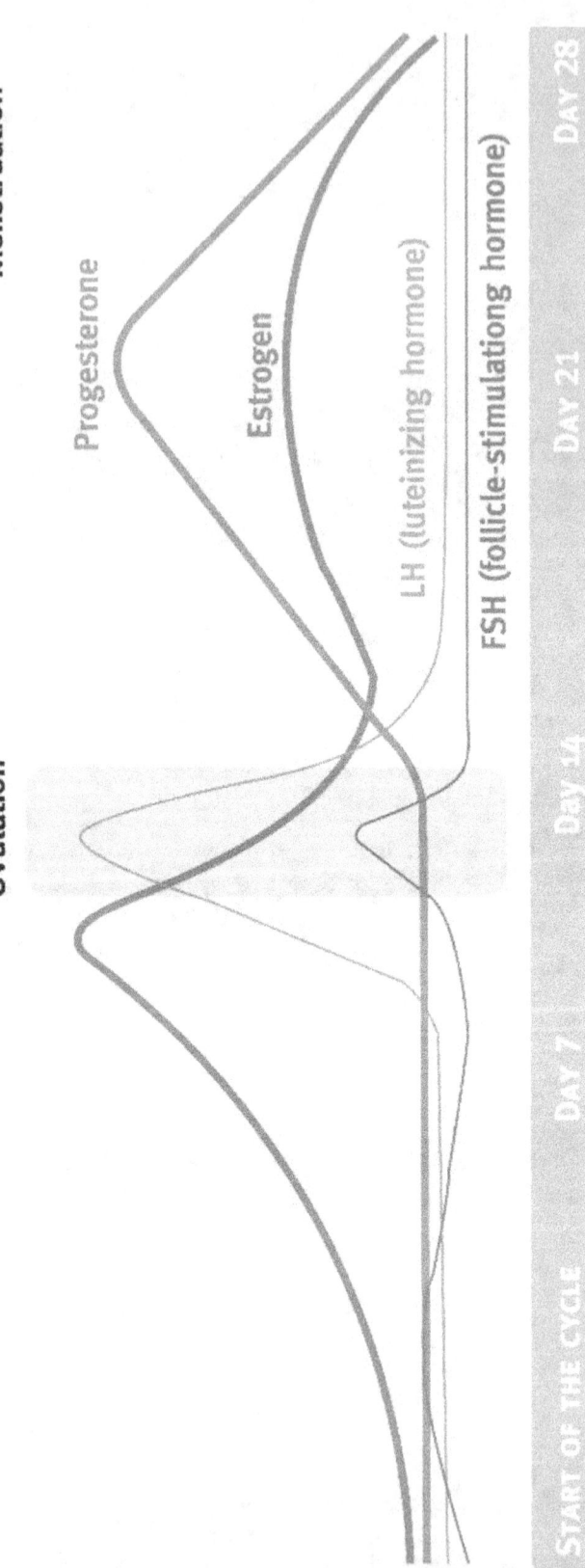

(3)

Estrogen

Estrogen is one of the most important hormones in the female body. It helps to regulate cholesterol, bone growth and muscle tissue. Released by the ovaries, this hormone is responsible for the female reproductive system, breast tissue growth, uterus lining, pubic and underarm hair, and menstruation. It is very active in the first 14 days of a woman's menstrual cycle or follicular stage. Estrogen plays a key role in boosting brain neurotransmitters, dopamine, serotonin, and GABA, referred to as our "pleasure center" or "feel good, sleep well" zone. Dopamine controls the body's energy, excitement, motivation, feeling of enjoyment and pleasure center. It's the body's natural amphetamine. Serotonin is a natural mood stabilizer promoting sleep, relaxation, calmness and a tranquil sense of wellbeing. GABA (gamma-aminobutyric acid) has a natural Valium effect on the body, counteracting anxiety, and bringing calmness to the body, mind, and spirit. Understanding how estrogen behaves in the female body will give you a better grasp on fat loss during the different stages of your menstrual cycle and during menopause.

Estrogen can also cause the body to store more fat tissue, especially in a woman's lower body. When a woman carries too much estrogen or becomes estrogen dominant, the body can respond with excessive weight gain, stubborn body fat storage (especially on the hips, butt and thighs), breast and uterine fibroids, irregular and/or heavy periods, fatigue, loss of sex drive, depression, or anxiety. Unfortunately, we live in an environment swarmed with estrogen-like toxins and chemicals known as "environmental estrogen," found in foods, plants, and a vast amount of commercial products we buy and use in our everyday lives. Some items that carry estrogen-like chemicals are water bottles and plastic containers, alcohol, cigarettes, drugs, refined sugars, food preservatives, caffeine, fast foods, cosmetics, personal care products, bacteria, viruses, mold, fungi, the air we breathe, food preservatives, heavy metals, radiation, petroleum, and many more as we continue to live in an environment of instant production and quick delivery using less expensive means. From this list, you can clearly see the problem this presents to a woman's fat loss program.

Progesterone

Progesterone is estrogen's counter partner in a woman's reproductive cycle, active in the last 14 days of menstrual cycle or luteal stage. This hormone triggers the lining of the uterus to thicken and prepare for the fertilized egg. Both estrogen and progesterone need to be in balance because they work collaboratively to regulate the female menstrual cycle. Too much, too little, or the absence of either will interrupt a woman's hormonal balance traumatically and most likely make weight management very difficult.

What is Estrogen Dominance?

Estrogen dominance refers to a relative deficiency of progesterone compared to estrogen.

- Stress negatively impacts progesterone; imbalance of estrogen and progesterone
- Environmental Estrogen Exposure (E.E.E.)
- Diet high in hormone injected foods (soy, meats, etc.)
- Fat Cells (fat cells aid in production of estrogen)
- Fibroids, fibrocystic breast, ovarian cysts, endometriosis

How to Lose Weight using the Menstrual Cycle

The first time I ever heard of the concept of losing weight working with my hormonal system (menstrual cycle), I was baffled. My trainer introduced me to Dr. Jade Teta's book, "Metabolic Effect," which inevitably helped me to loss over 40 pounds and keep it off.

In Dr. Teta's blog, "Exercise & Menstruation: Training with your cycle (Female Phase Training)," he exposes new concepts in the fat loss industry. This is cutting edge female technology! And guess what? It works! I've followed the protocol outline in his program and have lost a tremendous amount of body fat and helped my clients to do the same. Here's an excerpt:

> *"There are two distinct phases of the menstrual cycle. The follicular phase is marked by the beginning of menses (day 1 of the cycle) and ends at ovulation (day 14 of the cycle in the textbook case). It is called the follicular phase because the follicle (which contains the female egg) is maturing during this phase mainly under the influence of follicle stimulating hormone (FSH). The proper maturation of this follicle is essential for the release of an egg. The second phase of the cycle is the luteal phase. This phase is marked by ovulation and the subsequent transformation of the follicle into the corpus luteum once the egg is released. This phase is triggered by a large surge in lutenizing hormone which causes the follicle to "pop" and release its egg. The corpus luteum becomes the major source of progesterone. If the egg is not fertilized, the corpus luteum degrades, estrogen and progesterone levels both fall and the uterine lining is shed resulting in menses...Estrogen opposes insulin's action on the fat storing enzyme lipoprotein lipase (LPL), essentially making the body more insulin sensitive. The overall impact of estrogen is less fat storage and enhanced fat burning.*

"Estrogen is also anti-cortisol (as is progesterone). Given these considerations, the follicular phase of the menstrual cycle allows a greater tolerance for insulin promoting foods (starchy/fatty foods). It also makes the body more resistant to catabolic exercise modalities that may waste muscle, like long duration cardio... The follicular phase of the menstrual cycle is a great time to focus more on steady state longer duration moderate intensity cardiovascular exercise and heavy traditional weight training. This combination will enhance fat loss, and maintain or perhaps even gain lean muscle. Women will be able to burn higher amounts of fat and be less prone to muscle loss due to the estrogen effect during this time. Some research also hints the early follicular phase may produce the best performance outcomes for athletic women... Progesterone opposes the action of estrogen and may make the body more insulin resistant resulting in a greater propensity to store fat and lose muscle (5). Based on these metabolic considerations, women would want to watch their starch/sugar intake during the luteal phase and minimize more catabolic forms of exercise . With progesterone relatively higher than estrogen in the luteal phase, the female metabolism is more reliant on sugar versus fat metabolism... This metabolic state is more reminiscent of the male physiology and there is enhanced glycogen storage and a potential increased after burn from exercise (6). These luteal phase changes create a great opportunity to use higher intensity short duration metabolic conditioning (high rep weight training) and/or interval training (2, 4). By keeping the sessions shorter and more intense and using high rep weight training, perhaps we can overcome the slowed fat loss during exercise and keep exercise stress under control. This may maximize the hormonal responses, elevate fat loss and minimize muscle loss." (Dr. Jade Teta, 2013)

What does this have to do with fat loss?

In addition to having reproductive functions, estrogen and progesterone have an impact on fuel storage and fuel use. In other words, these two hormones can determine the type of fuel burned (sugar versus fat). This is mainly because they can mildly influence two primary fuels regulating hormones, insulin and cortisol.

What You Need To Know about Menopause

Night sweats! Anxiety! Moods! Lowered libido! Irritable all the time! And on and on... Welcome to MENOPAUSE! So, I decided to include a section in this book on menopause because if you are blessed to be over 40 years old, you are gonna experience it whether you want to or not. Menopause affects weight loss or will cause you to get fat -- if you don't know how to deal with it.

So what is menopause? Menopause is the normal biological process in women when the ovaries stop producing estrogen and progesterone and her menstrual cycle ceases. According the National Institute of Aging, there are 3 parts to menopause: *perimenopause* (several years before last menstrual period), *menopause* (the end of the menstrual cycle), and *post-menopause* (lasting the rest of your life). The age at which this occurs varies, but typically occurs from the mid to late 40s and early 50s.

Common symptoms of menopause are:
- Hot flashes, mood swings
- Tired, irritable
- Sleep, night sweats
- Bladder infections
- Sex drive
- Drier vaginal walls
- Osteoporosis
- Heart disease
- Stiffer joints and muscles
- Lose muscle, gain fat
- Belly fat
- Thinner skin

Heart disease and osteoporosis are common problems that can start at menopause. According to the American Heart Association, menopause doesn't cause heart disease, but certain risk factors increase during menopause, such as high-fat diets and smoking, and unhealthy habits adopted early in life begin to take a toll on the body. Estrogen helps to control bone loss and estrogen reduction, which certainly contribute to osteoporosis. For most women, over time these symptoms will go away without treatment. There are some cases where women may opt for hormone therapy to help manage the effects of hormonal imbalance. There are several natural remedies that assist with hormonal imbalance for women in menopause. Some of the best and most highly recommended natural remedies to ease menopause symptoms are:

- Maintain a balanced hormonal system
- Lower stress, cortisol, and estrogen levels
- Eat foods high in protein, low in carbohydrates
- Exercise smarter and better
- Reduce environmental estrogen exposure
- Ingest maca roots (see herb and spices section)

> *Cocoa Powder (ingredient in most dark chocolates), Maca root (increase energy, stamina, focus and believed to help boost estrogen levels), calming herbs and teas with chamomile, passionflower, skullcap, cinnamon bark, ashwagandha root, valerian root, and other soothing tea blends.*

Have you ever wondered why you get the urge for sweets, chocolate, or your favorite dish? During the last 14 days of the menstrual cycle (the luteal stage), estrogen and progesterone drop dramatically, which in turn produces a wide range of subdued symptoms. When a woman's estrogen is low, her ability to boost serotonin, dopamine, and GABA becomes an issue. Ultimately, the nervous system is affected, manifesting in mood swings, food cravings, irritability, depression, restlessness, anxiety, disorganization, fatigue, low libido, isolation, dreaded feelings, etc.

Gut Hormones and Fat Loss

On the following pages is a list of some gut hormones (as identified by the National Center for BioTechnology Information, NCBI) found in the human body that may play a role in fat loss.

Cholecystokinin (CCK)
CCK is responsible for stimulating the digestion or breakdown of fats and proteins in the body. According to NCBI, CCK is one of the first gut hormones that affects appetite. It is produced in the duodenum which is located between the stomach and small intestine. Producing more CCK has been shown to reduce appetite, therefore as one eats more protein, fiber, and healthy fat, it may facilitate fat loss.

Peptide (PYY)
PYY is produced in the intestines and colon, and acts to reduce appetite and obesity.

Neuropeptide Y (NPY)

NPY acts like a neurotransmitter produced by the brain and nervous system. Its main role is to stimulate appetite and store energy as fat. During times of stress, this hormone is elevated, which can lead to overeating, obesity, abdominal fat, etc.

There are several other gut hormones associated with appetite regulation such as GLP-1, oxyntomodulin, amylin, and pancreatic polypeptide. Some other important hormones associated with mood, exercise, and fat loss are hGH, DHEA, and testosterone.

Growth Hormone (hGH)

Human growth hormone is secreted by the pituitary gland. This hormone is primarily known to promote growth in children and adolescents, but also has various important metabolic functions throughout adult life ("Growth Hormone," NCBI, 2010). It also helps to build muscle, burn fat, and regulate body composition, body fluids, bone growth, sugar, fat metabolism, and a host of other health benefits. hGH is also referred to as the "fountain of youth." As one ages, especially beginning in their 30s, hGH production drops dramatically! Therefore, you must be proactive to help keep this powerhouse producing. Imagine having the physiological benefits of a growing and developing teenager, yet you are in your 40s, 50s, 60s, or 70s?

How to Increase hGH Naturally

Women who are pre-menopausal and perimenopausal want this powerhouse hormone on deck at all times. And I'm going to tell you plain and simple how to get it naturally and keep it cranking.

GO LIFT! Do not be afraid of weights! In fact, they will enhance your fat loss greatly. Deadlifts, bench press, pull-ups, bent rows, and squats, to name a few, are at the top of the list. When a person lifts heavier loads with the least amount of rest time, he or she causes the greatest amount of hGH to be released.

Do sprints. Because hGH releases from the pituitary gland in a pulsating fashion, when you do sprints, they allow for a very beneficial release of hGH because of the high lactic acid build up. Hence that young, tight, lean look!

Lastly, you gotta rest -- get plenty of sleep! Go to bed timely and get at least a solid 8 hours of rest. Human growth hormone production peaks significantly in the first few hours of sleep and continues throughout the night. Keep your sleep area dark and quiet. There is plenty of hype, bad research, and misdirection regarding growth hormone injection. Any mention of hGH in this book refers specifically to its natural production in the human body, not supplements or injection.

DHEA
Dehydroepiandrosterone (DHEA) is a natural steroid hormone produced by the adrenal gland. In the female body this hormone can convert to an androgen such as testosterone. It helps produce lean muscle tissue, improves bone density, boosts fat loss, increases libido, improves heart function, decreases risk of diabetes, and lowers inflammation.

DHEA is very important to produce in pre-menopausal and menopausal women because when the female organs stop producing estrogen and progesterone, DHEA, testosterone, and hGH become key hormones to manage weight.

Testosterone
In women, testosterone is produced primarily by the ovaries, adrenal glands and in peripheral tissue. Testosterone (an androgen known for the development of male characteristics and reproductive organs) plays a major role in a woman's muscle development, sex drive, and maintenance or repair of reproductive organs. Testosterone also is an anabolic (building) steroid naturally produced in the body. Women over 40 years old produce half the level of testosterone that women in their 20s produce. Testosterone is also important for a woman's libido or sex drive.

Average levels of testosterone in men compared to women:
Male:300-1,000 ng/dL
Female: 15-70ng/dL
(ng/dL = nanograms per deciliter)
Source: National Institutes of Health

One of the biggest problems women have with resistance training or lifting weights is the fear of bulking up and looking like a man. Testosterone, as mentioned, helps build muscle in a woman. Outside of steroid injection shots of testosterone, it is virtually impossible for a woman to ever put on the muscularity of a man when relying on the natural production and average levels of testosterone in a woman.

It is important to get beyond the fear of resistance training or weight lifting because burning fat and keeping it off requires you to build lean muscle. Remember this: *Muscle is Metabolism!!* The more you pack on lean muscle, the higher your metabolism. You will burn calories virtually effortlessly at a higher rate during rest than a person who is sedentary, obese, inactive, etc.

Control Centers for Hormones

There are a number of major organs and glands (such as the brain, heart, hypothalamus, thyroid, pituitary gland, adrenal glands, liver, kidneys, muscles, ovaries, and testes) that have a tremendous impact on how hormones are produced and regulated. They help in the daily functioning of the body. Other organs also play a role, so do not belittle their involvement in bodily functions.

The Liver and Fat Loss

The Body's Natural Filtration System

One of the most important organs believed to impact weight loss is the liver. The liver's main role is to filter the blood coming from the digestive tract before distributing it to the rest of the body, and to eliminate waste products. It also changes the nutrients we ingest to substances the body can store as needed, detoxify chemicals, and break down drugs. The liver is a major metabolic tissue vital to life. Imagine the importance of *filtered blood*. The liver regulates blood sugar levels so it stays constant, metabolizes proteins and fat, and eliminates waste products. If this process is disrupted in any way because of a sluggish, congested liver, weight loss can become a problem. When the body can efficiently and effectively process nutrients to use and get rid of waste, the body can function optimally. So, you're probably wondering why you need to know about all these hormones. Any malfunction or high/low volume chemical production of hormones can wreak havoc on your body's metabolic system and hormonal balance, and can make fat loss difficult. Visit a medical practitioner to get your liver and blood checked. Inquire as to the best ways to cleanse and detoxify the liver safely. This can help you gain a better understanding of your health status before starting a weight loss program.

HOW TO FIX IT
Lose the weight!
Focus eating more of the right things & exercising smarter
Consume high protein and alkaline vegetables
High fiber diet and regular bowel movements help decrease estrogen exposure
Lift heavy weights (hGH and testosterone)
Estrogen contraceptives and hormone replacement

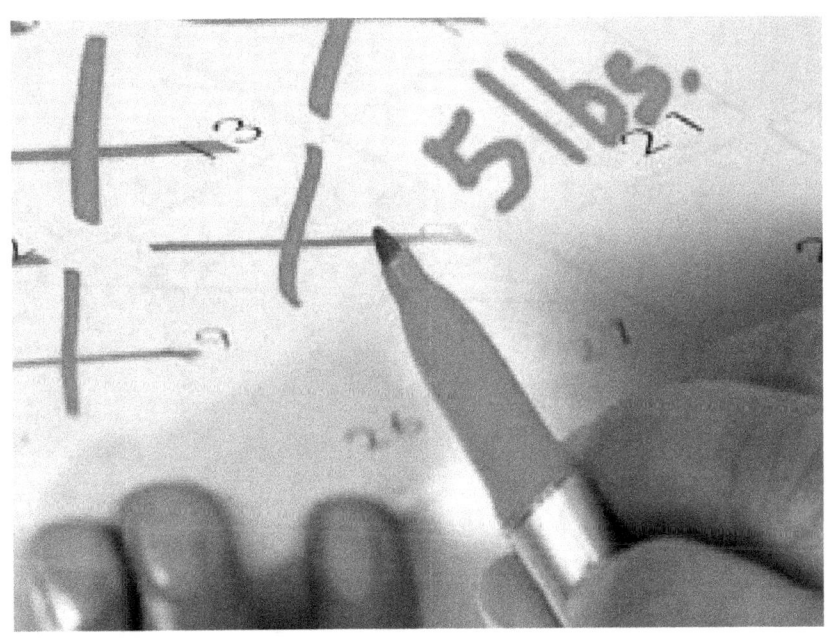

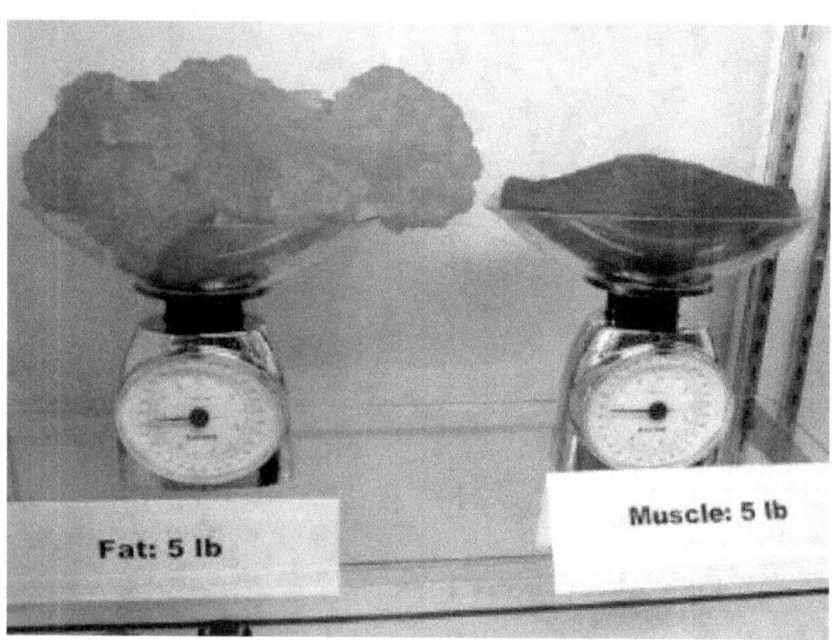

Which One Weighs More? Fat or Muscle?

(4)

Now, before you answer this question, think about it. Allow me to explain a few things about fat and muscle, first.

What is Fat?

Fat, the mushy, wiggly, sometimes unsightly blubber hanging in the wrong spots is simply adipose or loosely connected tissue located throughout the body. Fat can be found mainly between muscles under the skin, in the intestines, and around other organs including the heart. According to the American College of Sports and Medicine (ACSM), fat has a variety of functions needed for life.

Functions of Fat - Why we need it:
- Source of energy
- Provides the body insulation from extreme temperatures
- Cushions against concussive forces
- Satiety control (when eating healthy fats like olive oil, avocado oil, coconut oil, etc.)
- Gives food flavor
- Carries essential nutrients to the body like vitamin A, D, E, and K and other essential fatty acids

Here's the skinny on fat: The problem with fat occurs when there is too much of it stored in the body. Fat is a great source of energy the body can use, but as the body accumulates stored fat over the years through sedentary life style, poor diets, substantial weight gain, simply aging, etc., it will certainly open the door to a host of medical issues, diseases, and health complications. Ultimately, nobody wants to be fat, unsightly, and uncomfortable, constantly looking for bigger and bigger clothing, while heading down the road to unhealthy.

Are your organs fat?

A note on visceral fat and subcutaneous fat: One of the most dangerous places in the body for fat to be is lying directly next to your organs, which is known as visceral fat. According to National Center for Biotechnology Information (NCBI), *"The accumulation of fat around abdominal viscera and inside intraabdominal solid organs is strongly associated with obesity-related complications like Type 2 diabetes and coronary artery disease. The rate of visceral fat accumulation is also different according to the individual's gender and ethnic background; being more prominent in white men, African American women and Asian Indian and Japanese men and women."*

Abdominal obesity correlated closely with visceral and subcutaneous fat (located directly under the skin) is an excessive amount of fat located around the belly area, resembling the appearance of a "pot belly" or what many call a "beer belly." An individual carrying excess weight around the belly has an apple-shaped (or endomorphic) body type. Abdominal obesity is very harmful because, according to Harvard Medical School, *"Unlike subcutaneous fat, visceral fat cells release their metabolic products directly into the portal circulation, which carries blood straight to the liver. As a result, visceral fat cells that are enlarged and stuffed with excess triglycerides pour free fatty acids into the liver. Free fatty acids also accumulate in the pancreas, heart, and other organs. In all these locations, the free fatty acids accumulate in cells that are not engineered to store fat. The result is organ dysfunction, which produces impaired regulation of insulin, blood sugar, and cholesterol, as well as abnormal heart function."*

This is why developing a lifestyle of proper diet, exercise, and proactively addressing your current health status is critical to good health. The choice not to take action is the choice to subject your body to diseases that are preventable.

About that Muscle

"Cause I don't want to get bulky and look like a man..."

If there is to be any hope of losing weight, you will have to learn about and embrace muscle. Why? Muscle is metabolism. The section in this book on hormones should clear any doubt, fear, concern, or uncertainty about women getting bulky from lifting weights. Again, it is impossible for women to EVER look like a man from simply lifting weights to build healthy, lean, tone, fit, fat-burning muscle. God didn't create the female body to look like men. Only the use of steroids, or naturally skewed genetics or hormonal levels in some women, can lead to more masculine-like features.

So, what is muscle, then? Muscle is a band of fibrous tissue found throughout the body that is designed to contract, promote movement, and bring stability to body parts and positions. The more muscle you have, the higher your metabolism. For example, while you're resting, working on a computer, or sitting at home watching your favorite movie, your body's metabolism burns higher with increased muscle tissue than one who doesn't have as much muscle. According to a study conducted by NCBI, *"Energy expenditure varies among people, independent of body size and composition, and persons with a 'low' metabolic rate seem to be at higher risk of gaining weight. These findings suggest that differences in resting muscle metabolism account for part of the variance in metabolic rate among individuals and may play a role in the pathogenesis of obesity.*" In other words, the more muscle you have, the higher your metabolism, the more calories you burn at rest, which affects your BMR (Basal Metabolic Rate) and dictates the amount of energy/calories your body has to burn in order to maintain normal bodily functions.

Understanding Total Daily Energy Expenditure (TDEE)

How many calories do I burn in one day?

It's important to understand how the body burns calories/energy on a daily basis. When you have a better understanding of how the body uses energy, you will better grasp why you need to build the type of body that burns calories regularly with little to no effort so your body can function at optimal levels.

TDEE = Total Daily Energy Expenditure (BMR+NEAT+TEF+TEE)
BMR = Basal Metabolic Rate (65-70% of TDEE)
NEAT = Non-Exercise Activity Thermogenesis (15% OF TDEE)
TEF = Thermic Effect of Food (5-10% OF TDEE)
TEE = Thermic Effect of Exercise (5% of TDEE)

Total daily energy expenditure or (TDEE) is the number of calories/energy your body burns in a 24 hour period. TDEE is relative to each individual, therefore to find out what your TDEE is you can search the Internet for accurate formulas and equations (such as the Katch-McArdle equation, the Harris-Benedict, or the Mifflin-St Jeor equation) used in the industry to determine TDEE. If you are still uncertain how to approach finding an accurate measurement of your TDEE, visit your medical doctor, fitness professional, or nutritionist/dietician who can easily guide you through this process. For the sake of emphasis in this book, just know the definition of TDEE and you'll have the basics for getting a better understanding of maximizing your fat loss daily for the rest of your life!

Basal Metabolic Rate (BMR) is an important equation for fat loss because it is the minimal amount of energy a person expends at rest. Indicated by calories, it equates to about 65-70% of daily calories burned), including the functioning of heart, brains, lungs, muscles, other vital organs, and body systems (such as circulatory, digestve, nervous, etc.). The remaining percentage comes from other intentional intense activities like running, lifting weights, aerobics class, as well as daily regular/passive movement like walking, standing, housecleaning, carrying groceries, gardening, taking the steps, etc. The thermic effect (TEF) is the number of calories burned to process the foods you eat, which account for about 5-10% of your TDEE.

If you take a close look at the percentages, you should quickly identify a few components to best manipulate and increase your TDEE. One way would be to increase your BMR by adding more lean muscle mass. This tissue is highly metabolic, one of the largest most abundant tissues in the body and requires a lot of calories or energy to maintain it.

Consider also that there are only so many variables with BMR that can directly impact your heart, lungs, liver, brains, kidneys, etc. to increase BMR. Just note these organs burn a lot of calories collectively on a daily basis, but muscle is probably the easiest to manipulate. Learn more about muscle manipulation in the exercise section.

Another component you can use to manipulate TDEE is non-exercise activity (NEAT). Get out and move around, folks! Have you ever wondered how our predecessors from the 19th century to the baby boomers have managed to stay lean even though they didn't engage in all these 21st century exercises, fancy equipment, fad diets, etc.? Few had vehicles to drive and had to walk. The secret was they moved around alot! Sadly in today's society, media, telecommunication, peer pressure, and quick fixes like machines and body modifications, have encouraged laziness because everything is convenient. Who knows? Next you won't even have to get out of bed to go to the bathroom.

Older generations moved. They did gardening, carried groceries, cleaned around the house regularly, worked on the farm, operated equipment, rangled livestock, moved materials, and on and on. .See my point? Translate this to modern-day language…stop being lazy and incorporate more non-exercise activities into your daily routine -- park the car at the farthest end of the lot and walk instead of circling for a closer spot, walk a flight of stairs to the 2nd or 3rd floor instead of using the elevator, take frequent leisurely walks that are serene, tranquil, and relaxing (for stress, anxiety, and mental exhaustion), mow the lawn, pick up boxes (be sure to bend at the knees when lifting) one by one and carry them up or down the stairs, walk the dog, drop the car off at park and ride, take the train and walk the harbor, downtown, or scenic resorts. I think you get my point. Just MOVE!

Now, you're probably wondering what in the world this scientific language has to do with weight loss. As highlighted throughout this book, the importance of understanding how your body operates and the kinds of fuels/food/energy it needs to function will help to facilitate a successful fat loss program. Knowing how to take better care of your body for optimal functioning and effortless fat burning to keep lean muscle, will take you light years past most individuals who are still trying to lose weight the old fashion way (endless cardio, starvation diets, shots, pills, etc.). When you learn to choose the foods that are best for your body, you will know what nutrients are in the foods you eat and how they affect your overall performance and facilitate keeping a lean tone fit body for life -- then you will appreciate spending some time reading, learning, and applying the best tools for better health and wellness.

Why you really need muscle more than fat:

Body motion and movement like standing, sitting, walking and other physical tasks
Characteristics of extensibility, elasticity, excitability, contractibility and relaxation
Joint mobility and support
Balance and coordination
Support movements such as speed, power, endurance, and strength
Push, pull, and lift functionality

Now that you have a better understanding of the roles for fat and muscle, which one weighs more, fat or muscle? Take a look at this photo:

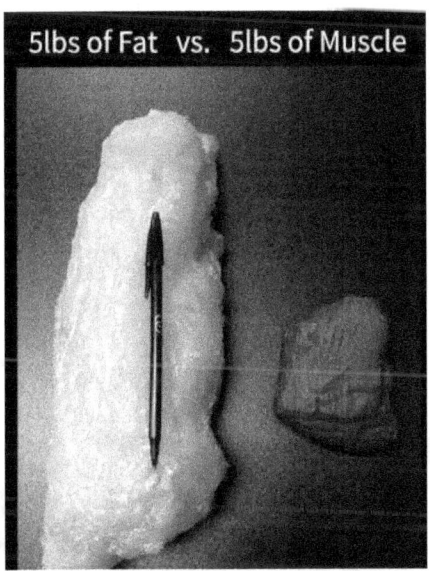

5lbs of Fat vs. 5lbs of Muscle

The answer to this question is simple: *Neither!* Muscle does not weigh more than fat nor does fat weigh more than muscle. The differentiating factor is the *amount of space* they take up in the body. Muscle is denser than fat which means two people can be the same height and weight but the person with a higher body fat percentage will wear larger clothing, look bigger, and be proportionately much different from the person who is smaller, carrying lean muscle, and wearing a smaller size.

Now, if you are comparing the same *portion size of fat* vs. *portion size of muscle,* then muscle would weigh more in this equation. Why? Muscle is denser (more compact) than fat and many muscle fibers can be stored in one place. This is why some women's body composition allows them to "carry their weight well," meaning if she is 5'5, 175 pounds, wears a size 10 with no medical diagnosis, and BMI is in the normal health range (under 25%), then chances are she is carrying more muscle than fat.

Muscle's Basket of Benefits

- Stronger muscles equals better performance
- Strong core is better able to support body weight
- Increases the number and size of calorie-torching muscle fibers
- Stronger muscles better hold joints in position
- Trains bones and builds new bone cells
- Makes bones stronger and denser, decreasing susceptibility to osteoporosis
- Strength training is cardio
- Decreases stress levels
- Weight control
- Reduced injuries
- Improved quality of life

Can I exchange my body fat for muscle?

This is a very common myth. The quick and easy answer is "NO!" Muscle and fat have distinctly different tissue and the process of how they are made makes it impossible for one to convert to the other.

Cellulite, those Annoying Dimples

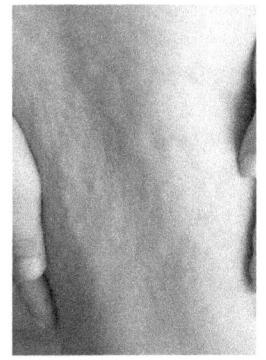 What are those annoying dimples on and around my hips, butt, and thighs? How many creams, lotions, devices, or surgery have you contemplated to get rid of those nasty little dimples sagging around various body parts? Cellulite is simply fat deposits located beneath the skin. One of the main symptoms of cellulite is the obvious appearance of lumpy, dimpled flesh mainly around the hips, buttocks, and thighs areas.

According to Dr. Jade Teta, in "Metabolic Effect," *"Women tend to carry increased body fat in the lower body, mainly because of the influence of estrogen, which increases the alpha-adrenergic receptor density in the butt, hip and thigh region. In addition, the vertical position of female collagen fibers results in fat cell accumulation inside 'collagen pockets.' This causes the characteristic dimpling and puckering of cellulite. Together these physiological characteristics can result in slow fat release from the lower body and/or issues with cellulite in both overweight and thin women."*

Dr. Teta did a fantastic job explaining the different receptors women have in their lower body, and how exercise, eating, and the right protocol can help decrease or remove cellulite from these areas.

> *"The catecholamines are the major drivers of fat loss during exercise. There are two types of receptors the catecholamines bind: alpha-adrenergic receptors and beta-adrenergic receptors. Think of the beta receptors as the fat burners (B for burn) and the alpha-receptors as slowing fat release (A for anti-burn). Because women have nine times more alpha compared to beta receptors in their lower body, they do not burn fat effectively from this area. In order to attack this we want to: 1) Block the alpha-receptors and 2) Ramp up beta-receptor stimulation. There are few ways to block the action of alpha-receptors. A 'low-carb' is the best way to reduce alpha-adrenergic receptor activity. The natural agent yohimbine also does this. A short, intense burst of activity can create a large catecholamine surge. With the alpha-receptors blocked, more fat can be released. To ensure all the released fat is burned, intense workouts followed by low intensity, long duration steady-state activities, like walking, are best."*

"There is little to impact the collagen aspect of the problem. Newer medical spa treatments that involve varying forms of mechanical massage, 'laser' light, heat, suction and pressure are MAY have benefit. Foam rolling and hydrotherapy, forms of self-guided deep tissue massage and blood flow stimulation, MAY also be beneficial. Coleus forskoli (forskolin) and Green Tea Extract (EGCG) can help reduce fat under low insulin environments. They work through mechanisms similar to the catecholamine hormones, but bypass the adrenergic receptor issue." (Teta, 2016).

How Much Fat Am I Carrying Around?

BMI Body Composition and Other Measurements

Have you ever visited the gym and spoken to a personal trainer, and he asks you when you last had your BMI checked? BMI (Body Mass Index) is a measurement that takes into account your weight relative to your height. According to ACSM, BMI is to body fat as height is to weight when determining risk factors for obesity.

Assessing your BMI is a good way to determine risk factors for obesity because of its high correlation to weight. The downside to using BMI measurements is the inability to arrive at precise numbers for weight gain or loss. Also, BMI doesn't distinguish between fat weight and fat-free weight.

Other Techniques to Determine Body Composition according to ACSM:
- Waist-to-hip circumference measures weight circumference or perimeter of the waist
- Skin folds - calipers are used to take measurements up to nine different locations on the body (one of the more accurate ways to determine body fat percentage)
- BIA (bioelectrical impedance analysis) is a noninvasive way to assess body composition

U.S. Obesity Epidemic

According to the National Center for Health Statistics, in 2014 over 36% of U.S. adults were obese. That's over 118,500,000 obese people -- over one-third of the population of the United States.

Obesity is defined as having a BMI of 30 or higher. To start your fitness journey, before you know where you're going, you need to find out where you are. *How much do you weigh? Are you overweight/obese? Have you been diagnosed with a medical condition such as diabetes, high blood pressure, cholesterol, etc.?* In 2013, the American Medical Association (AMA) recognized obesity as a disease because it impairs bodily functions. This recognition was later refuted because the main criteria used for diagnosis was BMI of 30 or above, which does not differentiate between fat mass and fat-free mass. Did you know that the number one leading cause of death in the U.S. is heart disease (American Heart Association, AHA 2015)? The causes for heart disease include obesity, diabetes, high blood pressure, high cholesterol, alcohol use, cigarette smoking, poor diet, and genetics. Whether you agree or not, you need to consider your personal health and well-being. If you're overweight, obese, fat, out of shape, suffering with any medical conditions, etc., you don't need to validate the obvious. Simply put, use an appropriate basis for determining your health status and do something about it. If you are overweight (BMI 25-29.9), obese (BMI 30-39.9), or morbidly obese (40+), chance are high that you will develop one or all of the following ailments: cardiovascular disease, diabetes, high blood pressure, high cholesterol, etc. -- and that's a fact.

"Well, I was born with this risk..."

Modifiable and Non-modifiable Risk Factors

For years I used to make these statements, "It's in the family," "I was born with it," "I can't help what I inherited," "It's in my genes," and "Well, you gonna die from something," etc. These statements and so many others are excuses for why you won't take charge of your health and do something about it.

Age, race, gender, genetics, and family history are classified as risk factors (non-modifiable) that you can't control. Obesity, high blood pressure, diabetes, cholesterol, cigarette smoking, and a sedentary lifestyle are modifiable risk factors you can and should make every effort to control. One of the risk factors I wanted to highlight in this list is *sedentary lifestyle*. A sedentary lifestyle is one composed of regular inactivity, lack of exercise, routine sitting or lying down for extended periods of time, and expending little to no energy.

Reminds me of a little furry creature called a sloth...

What is a sloth? It moves only when necessary and even then very slowly. It sleeps 15-18 hours per day, does not attract attention, and is defenseless. It is lazy, maintaining a good habitat for other organisms to live off of, and it generally hangs out upside down on a tree.

Sloth's daily behavior:
- Idle, apathy, lazy, lounging, loafing, sluggish, shiftlessness
- Lack of ambition and resourcefulness
- Dallying (do something slowly)
- Inertia (lack of movement especially when wanted or needed)

Interestingly, in the scriptures the sloth is mentioned synonymously with some of our thoughts and behavior:

"Not slothful in business; fervent in spirit; serving the Lord."
Romans 12:11
"The desire of the slothful killeth him; for his hands refuse to labour."
Proverbs 21:25
"The way of the slothful man is as an hedge of thorns: but the way of the righteous is made plain."
Proverbs 15:19

Since Adam and Eve, God has given man a choice. We can choose to be proactive with our health and get active. We can chose to stop making excuses about what we can't do and take action on what you can and should do.

Join a gym, buddy up with a friend for accountability, or hire a personal trainer. GET ACTIVE and take control of your life!

Diet & Nutrition

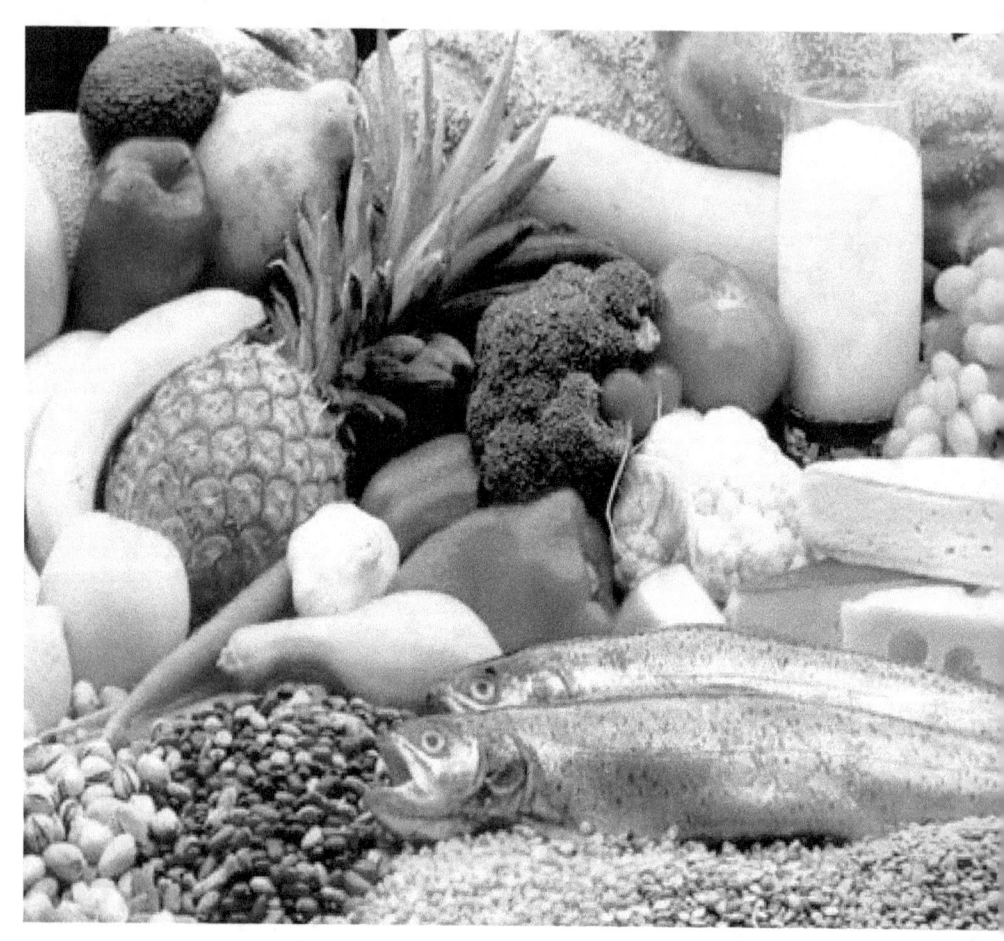

(5)

What kind of fuel (energy) are you putting in your body?

The word *diet* unfortunately has gotten a bad reputation for being a way to starve your body to weight loss. That's the general population view of a diet. Webster's dictionary defines a diet as, "food and drink regularly provided or consumed; habitual nourishment; the kind and amount of food prescribed for a person or animal for a special reason; a regimen of eating and drinking sparingly so as to reduce one's weight going on a diet." Diet and nutrition are synonymous and I want you to see that it's a *balance* of nutrient intake, not deprivation.

Please note: The following discussion on diet and nutrition are for general informational purposes only and not intended as a remedy or cure for anyone. There are no representations or warranties, express or implied, about the completeness, accuracy, reliability, suitability or availability with respect to the information, products, services, or related graphics, supplements or any discussion of foods or meal plan mentioned in this book. I am not a dietician, nutritionist, medical professor, or therapist. Please consult your primary physician before engaging in any exercise regimen, or strenuous physical activity, taking supplements, or changing your nutritional intake.

To get a better understanding of what foods to eat for fat loss, you need to understand what foods consist of (nutrients) and the role foods plays in your body. Nutrients such as carbohydrates, proteins, fats, vitamins, minerals, and water provide energy to the body and are essential for life. They should be consumed in balance to produce good health and overall body performance (ACSM). In this section, I will highlight the importance consuming quality foods with proteins, carbs, fat, and fiber in a way that helps you burn fat and build and/or keep lean muscle tissue.

Food for Fuel

Protein, carbs, and fats (macronutrients) are energy sources founds in foods, that provide the fuel the body needs. If your body gets the wrong fuel supply, too much, or none at all, the body's response can be impaired, dysfunctional, or it won't operate at all. A *calorie* is nothing more than a unit of measurement for energy in foods.

Did you know 3500 calories = 1 Pound

Caloric Content

Fat:	1 gram = 9 Calories
Protein:	1 gram = 4 Calories
Carbohydrates:	1 gram = 4 Calories
Fiber:	1 gram = 0-1 Calories

Muscle building Machine

Proteins are compounds composed of amino acids essential to many functions in the body, such as building muscle, balancing fluids, and producing enzymes for hormone production. They are also building blocks for skin, hair, bones, nails, and other connective tissue and can be used as a source of energy in the body. Protein quality is very important because the body can produce 11 non-essential amino acids, out of 20. The remaining 9 essential amino acids cannot be made in the body and must be provided through nutritional intake.

Foods such as tuna, chicken, crabmeat, turkey, salmon, beef, lamb, pork, cheese shrimp, and grains are good sources of protein. The important thing to remember about protein is you need to eat it with every meal. Protein is very filling (satiating) and highly thermic, which means it takes a lot of energy to break down this nutrient in the body for use. This process requires the use of calories (energy). For example, try eating 3 full chicken breasts for dinner and see how fast you can eat them and get full. Then, see how long you stay full.

The longer you stay full, the less you are likely to overeat. This could create a caloric deficit that can aid in fat loss. As I mentioned in the section on hormones, the goal is to ultimately balance your hormonal system, which is directly related to the foods you put in your body. Eating more protein can help create a caloric deficit which does not equate to depriving yourself of meals. Instead, eat foods that are filling, have a high thermic affect, nutritional, and help maintain hormonal balance. This is the perfect storm for weight loss.

Eating Carbs Make You Fat!

Wrong!!! Carbs have a terrible reputation for being foods that make you fat. Not so! Without this nutrient, your muscles' preferred source of energy, you will be sluggish, irritable, experience a sharp decrease in mental acuity, and have little or no energy to move a muscle.

Carbohydrates can come in two forms:

    1) Simple Carbohydrates: glucose, fructose, sucrose, maltose, galactose coming from foods like table sugar, milk, certain fruits and vegetables, grains, starch or gum, etc.

    2) Complex carbohydrates: polysaccharides (containing many molecules of sugar) such as starch, glycogen, cellulose from foods such as potatoes, spaghetti, beans, rice, oatmeal, wheat foods, etc. (ACSM)

Did you know that the sole source of energy for the brain is from carbs (glucose)? .According to NCBI, *"Glucose is virtually the sole fuel for the human brain, except during prolonged starvation. The brain lacks fuel stores and hence requires a continuous supply of glucose. It consumes about 120 g daily, which corresponds to an energy input of about 420 kcal (1760 kJ), accounting for some 60% of the utilization of glucose by the whole body in the resting state."*

Processed carbs and refined sugar are the worst carbohydrates to ingest. There is nothing beneficial about these types of carbs, though they store fat and create the perfect enironment in the body for diseases. Processed carbs and refined sugars include white bread, pasta, white sugar, candy, soft drinks, sugary beverages (including fruit juice), pretzels, chips, crackers, donuts, bagels, and white rice. They are also hidden in foods like mayonnaise, ketchup, sauces, glazes, canned foods, wheat products, and a host of other toppings and spreads we put on our foods.

Fiber is a carbohydrate the body can't digest so it has no calories. This nutrient can help with fat loss because it's satiating, decrease appetite, helps with regular bowel movement, and helps to keep blood sugar levels in check. This nutrient can be found in copious amount in foods like collard greens, broccoli, berries, avocados, artichokes, brussel sprouts, black beans, chickpeas, turnips, lentils, lima beans, chia seeds, flaxseed and other fruits, vegetables, nuts, andbeans, legumes which are rich in fiber.

Ultimately, for fat loss, women should find a balance with daily nutrition high in proteins, water, and fiber, low carbs, and healthy fat. A low carb lifestyle affords the body, especially in women over 30 years old, to burn fat in those tough areas and use it for fuel/energy instead of storing it. A sedentary lifestyle with a high fat diet, white starches, wheat bread (gluten), dairy, and excess carbs, dairy products, and excessive carbohydrate consumption will quickly move you into the obese column and could cause a host of diseases. The keys are balance and the right food choices!

Does eating fat make you fat?

Good Fat vs. Bad Fat Exposed!

Fat is not all bad! Fat has many vital functions for daily living. It is the body's preferred source of energy. However, you need to know if you are eating, saturated fat or unsaturated fat.

Saturated fats (triglycerides, diglycerides, and monoglycerides) are in foods like cheese, egg yolks, coconut oil, palm oils, butter, chicken/poultry, beef burgers, milk, nuts, seeds, lard, shortening, etc. These fats notably stay solid at room temperature and generally are derived from animals. These fats also tend to increase cholesterol in the body.

Unsaturated fats, which are mostly liquid at room temperature, can be polyunsaturated fats (high in vitamin E) which are good for reducing bad cholesterol. Monounsaturated fat lowers bad cholesterol while maintaining good cholesterol (ACSM).

Polyunsaturated Fats	Monounsaturated Fats
Fish Oil	Almonds, Pistachios, Brazilian, Hazelnut,
Vegetable Oil	Pecans, Macadamia Nuts
Corn Oil	Avocado Oil
Walnut Oil	Olive Oil
Hemp Oil	Peanuts
Canola Oil	High-oleic sunflower & safflower oil
Flaxseed Oil (high in omega 3's)	

Trans-Fats: The Worst Artery Cloggers

Trans-fats…the worst of fats. Don't pass go, don't collect $200, and go straight to the doctor's office for pills, shots, surgeries, and tactics for reducing high cholesterol, cardiovascular disease, stroke, diabetes, etc. Eating foods containing trans-fats will pave the road filled with these diseases.

Trans-fats occur naturally in animals (dairy and meats) or artificial (trans-fatty acids), which are created in an industrialized fashion. Trans-fats are used regularly in foods like vegetable shortening, margarine, crackers (even those that sound healthy), cereals, candy, baked goods, cookies, granola bars, chips, snack foods, salad dressings, fats, fried foods, popcorn, pie crusts, and many other processed foods labeled hydrogenated or partially hydrogenated.

Trans-fats were developed during the backlash against saturated fat -- artery-clogging animal fats found in butter, cream, and meats. Then food manufacturers realized that trans-fats lasted longer than butter without going bad. The result: Today trans-fats are found in 40% of the products on your supermarket shelves. A good way to remember what foods are loaded with trans-fats is to avoid all the food isles in the center of supermarket.

Zero Trans-Fats Doesn't Mean Zero Trans-Fats

Did you know that the Food Drug Administration (FDA) defines "zero trans-fats" as less than .5 gram per serving? This means the food you're eating out of the box that says "zero trans-fat" actually has trans-fats in every serving. So you may be consuming more trans-fats than you know. Stay away from hydrogenated oils, partially hydrogenated oils, and trans-fatty acids!

Damaging Effects of Eating Trans-fats
- bad cholesterol
- fat in blood
- insulin levels
- risk of cancer, diabetes, heart disease
- inflammation in the body
- chances of stroke
- plague build up in arteries

Note: Studies have shown there are a host of other negative effects that eating trans-fats have on the body's systems including cardiovascular, immune, and hepatic (liver) systems

---

According to World Health Organization (WHO), "*A growing number of countries in the WHO European Region have recognized that taking action to eliminate trans-fats may bring significant health gains, and new data indicate that such action is highly effective in reducing trans-fat consumption among the population. Europe now leads the world in the number of countries that have taken action to virtually eliminate trans-fats from our diets. If more countries act, the benefits to health can be substantial across the whole Region.*" (Zsuzsanna Jakab, WHO Regional Director for Europe)

In 2013, the U.S. FDA made a preliminary determination that PHOs (partially hydrogenated oils) were no longer "generally recognized as safe" (GRAS). FDA is finalizing that action and determining that PHOs are not GRAS for any use in human food.

> *"We made this determination based on the available scientific evidence and the findings of expert panels. Studies show that diet and nutrition play a key role in preventing chronic health problems, such as cardio vascular disease and today's action goes hand in hand with other FDA initiatives to improve the health of Americans, including updating the Nutrition Facts label." (Susan Mayne, Ph.D., Director of FDA's Center for Food Safety and Applied Nutrition).*

Trans-fat occurs naturally in meat and dairy products, so they can not be eliminated completely. They are also present at very low levels in other edible oils, where it is unavoidably produced during the manufacturing process. In addition, companies can petition FDA for specific uses of certain partially hydrogenated oils.

As you can see, there is clearly a distinction between good fat and bad fat. Yes, you can and should eat the good fat that is beneficial to the body. Eating good fat does not make you fat, however eating a diet high in saturated (bad) fats along with a load of carbs is the perfect storm for massive weight gain. Another key point to remember about good fats is that it is dense and high in calories so you don't need to eat a lot of it. Some studies have shown eating healthy fat such as coconut oil, olive oil, nut oils, flaxseed oil (which has the richest source Omega 3 fat), and fish oil can help with fat loss. Coconut oil, though a saturated fat (medium chain triglycerides, MCT), is especially noted to help with fat loss because of its fast absorption rate and its immediate availability for the body to use.

To lose the weight and stay in shape for life, you must remember to read your food labels and know what kinds of fats you're putting in your body. Avoid foods with added saturated fat. Avoid trans-fats, anything hydrogenated, partially hydrogenated, and trans-fatty acids at all costs! Be proactive, get educated, make better foods choices, and save your life.

Herbs, Wholefoods, and Super Foods

Dynamite foods for your body

Society is overrun with quick fixes to eat fast food, heavily processed foods, microwave dishes, etc. If you took a moment and glanced in your seasoning cabinet, you'll be amazed that some of the best natural healing foods are located in your kitchen -- and you only sprinkle them lightly, if at all, in your dishes. Herbs, wholefoods, and super 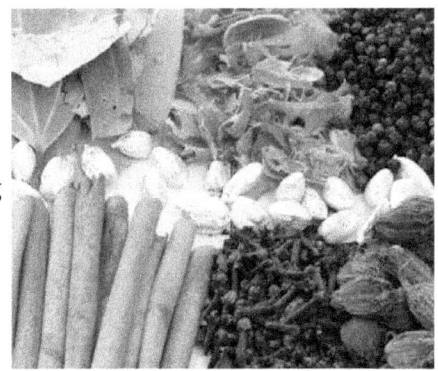 foods work interchangeably, but I wanted to share a few notes on these food choices that I believe are best for maintaining overall health, wellness, and for maintaining a healthy lifestyle.

Developing a lifestyle using herbs and spices can be a great start to your weight loss journey. Holistic healing, homeopathic, nutritional, drug free healing, and non-synthetic medical remedies can be beneficial. Herbs comes from the green or leafy part of plants. Spices, on the other hand, come from parts of the plant like the seed, bulb, stem, or root. The benefits of learning how to use these foods to enhance overall well-being, or even to cure some health issues, is well worth the investment.

According to Prescription for Nutritional Healing, *"In the United States, herbal remedies were widely used until the early 1900's when what was to become 'now known as' the modern pharmaceutical industry isolating compounds and producing drugs based on them. Over the years, most Americans have become conditioned to rely on synthetic, commercial drugs for relief. Today's renewed interest in herbs reflects increasing concern about the side effects of powerful synthetic drugs as well as the desire of many people to take charge of their own health rather than turning themselves over to a corporate health system."* The vast benefits of eating and using herbs and spices to heal your body of diseases, lose weight, prevent or cure aliments, and so much more, should warrant anyone to study this way of life further.

The following list includes some of the most powerful, healing, nutritional, and overall health and wellness-enhancing herbs and spices, many of which I'm sure are in your kitchen right now. Who knows, you may have been housing your own herbal and healing pharmacy in your kitchen and didn't know it.

Please note: This is not an exhaustive list of herbs and spices. There are too many plant sources to name that have nutritional and healing properties, and remedies for cures. Listed are some of the more popular ones found in the average kitchen and their health benefits. You must study these herbs and spices to get full spectrum of benefits.

Cinnamon - *diabetes, weight loss, warms the body, enhance digestion, yeast infection, fungal infection, good multi-vitamin source (calcium, chromium, copper, iodine, iron, magnesium, zinc, Vitamins A, B, C, etc.*

Ginger - *anti-inflammatory, clean colon, circulation, strong antioxidant, soothe stomach, reduce cramps, hot flashes, headache, muscle pain, good multi-vitamin source (magnesium, calcium, potassium, amino acids, iron, vitamins B, C, and many more.*

Parsley - *prevents tumors multiplying, stimulates digestive system, expels worm, relieve gas, freshen breath, helps bladder, kidney, stomach, thyroid functions, release fluid retention, obesity, vitamin C (contains more than oranges by weight) calcium, iron, magnesium, selenium, zinc, vitamins A, B, C, and E, etc.*

Basal - *protect blood vessel from free radical damage, may prevent cholesterol, heart attacks, strokes, anti-bacterial, vitamin K, manganese, calcium, vitamin A, C and more.*

Garlic - *detoxify body, immune system, improve circulation, cold, flu, calcium, folate, iron, potassium, zinc, selenium, and more.*

Turmeric - *fights free radicals, protects liver against toxins, aids circulation, lowers cholesterol, antibiotic, anticancer, anti-inflammatory, believe to prevent or treat Alzheimer's disease, calcium, iron, potassium, zinc, Vitamins B, C and more. NOTE: curcumin, the most active derivative of turmeric has shown to have many health benefits from strengthening the immune system to curing many diseases.*

Cayenne Pepper - *reduce inflammation, improve circulation, antiseptic, arthritis, alpha & beta carotene, amino acids, iron, folate, potassium, zinc and more.*

Thyme - *eliminates gas, reduce fever, headache, and mucus, asthma, bronchitis and other respiratory problems, strong antiseptic properties, lowers cholesterol, eliminates itchy, flaky scalp caused by candidiasis, good multi-vitamin source (too many to list).*

Fenugreek - *laxative, reduce fever, mucus, sinus problems, lower cholesterol, calcium, amino acids, fatty acids, iron, magnesium, selenium, zinc and more.*

Green Tea - *strong antioxidant, promising weight loss aid, anti-cancer, immune system, lower sugar, reduce blood clotting, good for asthma, combats mental fatigue, may delay onset of atherosclerosis, fights tooth decay, amino acids, calcium, iron magnesium, potassium, zinc, vitamins B, C and more.*

Celery - *reduce blood pressure, diuretic, antioxidant, relieves muscle spasms improves appetite, good multi vitamin source (too many to list).*

Chamomile - *reduce inflammation, stress, and anxiety, stimulate sleep, mouthwash for minor sores and gum infections, reduce fevers, headaches and pain, nerve tonic, choline, vitamins B, and C.*

Clove - *antiseptic, antiparasitic, digestive aid, toothache or mouth pain, calcium, iron, magnesium, potassium, zinc vitamins A, B, C and more.*

Flax seeds - *strong bones, nails, teeth, anti-inflammatory, female disorders, amino acids, calcium, essential fatty acids, iron, magnesium, sulfur, zinc, vitamins B, E, and more.*

Eucalyptus - *decongestant, antiseptic, colds, cough, respiratory issues.*

Golden Seal - *very powerful cleanser and cure, fights infection, clean body, build immune system, spleen, liver, colon, pancreas, lymphatic, respiratory systems, Use first sign of cold or flu can stop. Good for allergies, ulcers, disorders affecting the bladder, stomach, prostate or vagina, calcium, iron, selenium, potassium, zinc, phosphorus, magnesium, manganese*

Lavender - *relieves stress and depression, good for burns, headaches, psoriasis.*

Lemongrass - *astringent, tonic, digestive aid, useful for fever, flu, headaches, calcium, iron, manganese, magnesium, zinc, selenium, etc.*

Olive Leaf - *good for virtually any infectious disease, fights against bacteria, viruses, fungi, antioxidant, potential lower blood pressure, good for viral infections, arthritis, helps stave cold and flu, calcium.*

Dill - *protect against free radicals, anticancer, antibacterial, calcium, manganese, vitamin C, and more.*

Mustard seed - *improve digestion, aids in metabolism of fat, applied externally helpful for chest congestion, joint pain, inflammation, injuries.*

Peppermint - *increase stomach acidity, aid digestions, anesthetized mucus membrane and the gastrointestinal tract, useful for rheumatism, chills, colic, diarrhea, headaches, heart trouble, nausea, poor appetite, calcium, choline, iron, potassium, vitamins B, E, and more.*

Maca - *increase energy and supports immune system, good for anemia, chronic fatigue, menopausal symptoms and menstrual problems, amino acid, calcium, iron, zinc magnesium, phosphorus, vitamins B, C, E, and more. Other known herbs and spices in the kitchen: Onion powder, chili powder, paprika, bay leaf, sea salt, vanilla extract, tarragon, cilantro.*

Curry powder - *reduce inflammation, anticancer, aids digestion, asthma, bronchitis, brain boosting compounds, believe to protects against Alzheimer's disease.*

Black Pepper - *improve digestion, prevents gas, promote intestinal health, sweating, urination, antibacterial, antioxidant, stays appetite, stimulates the breakdown of fat cells, magnesium, Vitamin K, copper, fiber, calcium, chromium and more.*

Rosemary - *fights free radicals, inflammation, bacteria, fungi, stimulates circulation, acts as astringent and decongestant, detoxify liver, anticancer, antitumor, lower blood pressure, good for menstrual cramps, calcium, iron, potassium, magnesium, zinc, vitamin B, C, and more.*

Sage - *stimulates central nervous system, digestive tract, reduce sweating, hot flashes, estrogen deficiency, whether menopause or following hysterectomy, used to dry up milk when women wish to stop nursing, boron, calcium, iron magnesium, phosphorus, selenium, zinc, vitamins B, C, and more.*

Oregano - *fights free radicals, inflammation, bacterial, viral and fungal infections, boost immune system, menstrual irregularities, fatigue, eczema, sinusitis, digestive problems, bronchitis, chronic infections, calcium, essential fatty acids, iron, magnesium, potassium, etc.*

Cumin - *excellent source of iron, controls diabetes, aids digestion, build immune system, anticancer, magnesium, copper, calcium, and more.*

Source: "Prescription from Nutritional Healing" 3rd Edition, WorldsHealthiestFoods.org

Wholefoods: The Better Food Selection

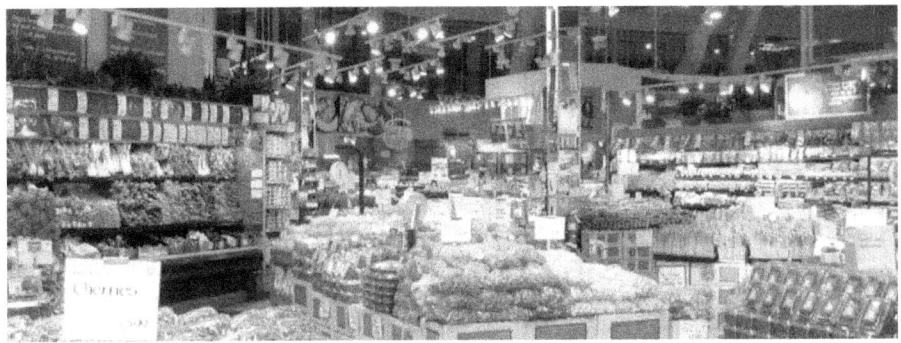

If you ever want to lose weight and keep it off effortlessly then you need to get acquainted with wholefoods. They are easy on digestion, absorption, and they are ready-made fuel for the body. Wholefoods are free of additives, artificial substances, and any man-made additions. These foods are unrefined and have minimal (if any) factory processing. The goal is to find and eat the best foods for your body that have not been tampered with or that have little added to intensify flavor, taste, appearance, quantity, etc.

Some examples of whole foods are apples, oranges, watermelon, bananas, grapes, peaches, yams, kale, carrots, collards, squash, eggplant, tomatoes, and almost any fruit or vegetable you can think of grown naturally from a seed. Though there is much discussion on genetically modified organisms (GMO), foods grown in a laboratory, for the purposes of this book we'll conclude you are already purchasing foods from vetted groceries stores, like Trader Joe's, Whole Foods, MOMS, local farmers markets, which generally disclose the sources of their produce. If you grow your food yourself, even better.

The majority of mainstream supermarkets are overrun with overpriced produce and foods that are loaded with chemicals and preservatives, and highly-refined processed laboratory-created hybrids that look good and taste good. These foods also are loaded with additives designed to keep you buying it over and over again to get that same taste and feel every time.

Have you ever noticed how you always have to get the extra-large container of hazelnut creamer, the super-sized box of salted crackers, 5 different flavors of your favorite 100% juice, and assorted boxes of cereal? Producers of these products know exactly what to put in the hottest selling food items to keep you buying it and eating it until you get addicted, fatter and fatter, and so sick you have to rely on medications to function daily.

Go Organic and Pay for It! NO EXCUSES!

Wholefoods and organic foods are synonymous in the health and wellness industry so here's the skinny on whether or not to buy organic. Buy organic every chance you get. Again, there is still ongoing industry discussion about organic foods being GMO's, imported foods loaded with pesticides, herbicides, and other harmful chemicals to preserve freshness. Lately in the news, a well-known herbicide used around the world, Round Up (herbicide chemical used on crops), has been on the hot seat for its known damaging effects to humans. According to the Environmental Protection Agency (EPA), under President Donald Trump, Administrator Scott Pruitt refuses to ban the use of widely-used pesticide despite scientific recommendations from his own agency that this pesticide has been linked to learning disabilities. In March 2017, Scott Pruitt signed an order denying a petition that sought to ban chlorpyrifos, a pesticide crucial to U.S. agriculture which is found in Round Up. When you read news that clearly demonstrates detriment and harm to your body, there remains no other choice but to be proactive and choose better food selections, or subject you and your family to deadly foods.

Probably one of the best ways (not the only way) to keep sane and buy the right foods for your health is to get in touch with your local farmers. Talk with them, ask question about where and how they grow their foods. Most farmers will be happy to tell you and back it up by inviting you to their local farms. Yes, you can get to the farm probably less than a few hours and get your food delivered to you, fresh! Most local farmers are very well versed about their industry, and they want to educate and keep you informed. They want your business and referrals. Believe me, no farmer wants a bad reputation because false advertisements say their foods are not grown naturally as they claim. They'll probably be out of business within 24 hours. That's just how fast news travel in the holistic, homeopathic, naturally-grown produce and livestock industry.

There is also a list of foods you don't necessarily have to buy organic.

To follow is a list of some foods you should buy organic. This list is not exhaustive and constantly changes as new research is conducted. The best rule of thumb is that most foods with a thick, hard outer covering can be bought non-organic. Foods with thin, soft, pealable skin you eat along with inner substance, you should buy organic. These are generally loaded with pesticides and can carry as much as 60 or more chemical on its outer layer to preserve some level of fresh appearance until it is purchased. Always wash all fruits and vegetables thoroughly before consuming them, even the thick-skinned foods.

Foods you should by organic (foods with the highest level of pesticides):
Nectarines
Grapes
Cucumbers
Tomatoes
Potatoes
Summer Squash
Apples
Spinach
Bell Peppers
Hot Peppers
Strawberries, Blueberries, Raspberries, Blackberries
Leafy Greens
Peaches
Celery
Meats: organic grass fed animal, natural, free range, or wild
Check with your local farmers markets

Foods you do not need to buy organic (foods with the lowest pesticide load);
Avocados
Sweet corn
Pineapples
Cabbage
Sweet peas (frozen)
Onions
Asparagus
Mangoes
Papayas
Kiwi
Eggplant
Grapefruit
Cantaloupe (domestic)
Cauliflower
Sweet potatoes
Coconut, lemons, limes, bananas, oranges

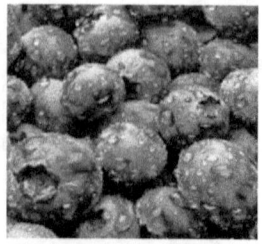

The next time you go grocery shopping, look for the foods with a little red cape on the backside. Okay, maybe not, but the foods that fight for you 24/7 are the ones you want to buy. Super foods is often synonymous with antioxidants, that are very rich in nutritional value and carry massive benefits for overall health and well-being. Onions, garlic, bell peppers, green leafy vegetables, teas, flaxseeds, brussel sprouts, broccoli, cabbage, beans, herbs, cocoa powder, red wine, nuts, seeds, berries family (especially blueberries) are some examples. These foods carry many benefits for your overall health and in some instances acts like white blood cells fighting off inflammation, infections, disease, etc.

Though preventive health care sounds like a misnomer or cliché, in this modern-day society, you need to consider moving your health care from a system designed to keep you sick by treating the symptoms, to an individual who will keep your best health interest and longevity at the forefront. That person is you! In other words, learn how to fight off diseases and preventing them all together by using the right and best foods, thereby creating a condition in the body where oxidants or free radicals can't survive. Better to set up and secure your fortress before the enemy arrives, than to let him walk right up to the drawbridge and come in at will, stealing and destroying everything in his way. Once he's finished causing major damage killing whomever and whatever is left, he takes over the fortress and invites his comrades, who are worse than him. You see the analogy here? When you don't do the things necessary to take care of your God-given vessel and live haphazardly, you leave the door open for diabetes, high blood pressure, high cholesterol, heart disease, stroke, and so many other diseases that will eventually destroy your body.

Inflammation, Weight Loss, and Health

The Secret Silent Killer

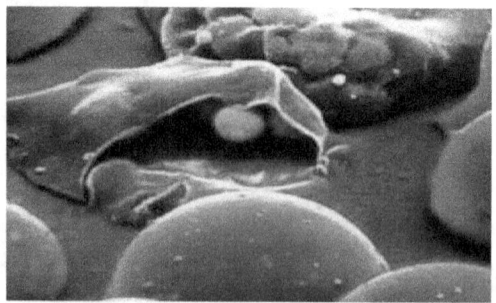

Listen up. This is probably one of the most important sections in this book. When you hear the word "inflammation," it may bring to mind a cut on the finger that swells up, turns red, hurts, and bleeds, or a sprained wrist, knee, or ankle that begins to swell, hurt, and maybe have its own heartbeat. Well, you're right! Inflammation is the body's defense mechanism, a natural response from the immune system designed to bring back homeostasis or balance to the injury before inflammation can occur.

According to the Free Dictionary, *"Inflammation is localized protective response elicited by injury or destruction of tissues, which serves to destroy, dilute, or wall off both the injurious agent and the injured tissue. The classic signs of inflammation are heat, redness, swelling, pain, and loss of function. An inflammatory response can be provoked by physical, chemical, and biologic agents, including mechanical trauma, exposure to excessive amounts of sunlight, x-rays and radioactive materials, corrosive chemicals, extremes of heat and cold, or by infectious agents such as bacteria, viruses, and other pathogenic microorganisms. Although these infectious agents can produce inflammation, infection and inflammation are not synonymous."*

Foreign Agents in your Body

"Why you stressing girl?"

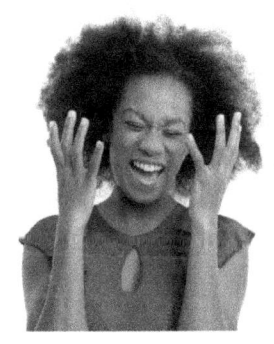

Did you know the inside of your body can become inflamed from ingesting foods with sugary, salty, starchy, greasy, fried, fattycontent and no nutritional value? Did you know that lack of exercise, stress, anxiety, worrying, anger, lack of sleep, alcohol, the presence of oxidants, toxins, imbalanced PH, and free radicals floating around in your blood also provokes inflammation? According to Dr. Johnny Bowden, Ph.D, holistic nutritionist, stress is the most inflammatory non-food causing illness and diseases. Chronic inflammation, alkaline/acidic imbalance, oxidative stress, anger, and unchecked emotions can damage the immune system and make you sick. The consequences of inflammation in the body are clinical depression, heart disease, diabetes, high blood pressure, high cholesterol, cancer, Alzheimer's disease, obesity, anxiety attacks, autoimmune diseases, arthritis, and bone issues. The important point to remember is that when any part of your body lacks oxygen, it dies. Starve your blood cells and death of internal organs, tissue, and the entire body is the end result. When cellular death occurs, health issues such as heart attack, stroke, cancer, organ failure, poor blood circulation, amputation, and many more can result.

So, STOP STRESSING! Learn to prioritize your life, putting family, friends, school, job, church, people, places, and other things in balance and proper perspective so that you control your boundaries. Proverbs 4:23 tells us, *"Keep thy heart with all diligence; for out of it are the issues of life."*

Weight Loss Quickie Expedition

The Truth about Fad Diets, B12 Shots, Wraps, Creams, Surgery, Weight Loss Pills, Fancy Equipment, and the Next Weight Loss Invention Tool

I would be remiss if I don't mention the hype about quick weight loss using the latest piece of equipment, pill, or diet. To set the record straight, if you're not willing to take pills or shots, have surgeries, use starvation diets and tight pieces of clothing the rest of your life, then don't start out with it. The majority of these items sold on the market are gimmicks, scams, and short term solutions to a long standing problem with your thinking. Nobody wants to put forth the time, energy, effort, work, or commitment it takes to be healthy. Instead, we want to get it overnight.

Now think for a moment, did you get fat overnight or was it a steady progression and lifestyle of poor eating habits, bad food choices, lack of exercise, not giving the proper attention your health and wellness needs on a daily basis? If you're honest, you might admit that you've psychologically adopted a lifestyle of neglect, passivity, and quick fixes to almost any problem including your health. And now the doctor is telling you, unless you correct the problem, you're heading for a metabolic storm and a disease-infested body. This may sting a bit, but honesty is the best policy, and truthfully, the final choice is yours.

The best tool you can use, not buy, is the matter between your two ears. Yes, your brain. Nothing will help you lose weight until you fix your faulty thinking and belief systems about health, wellness, and the need to be proactive (not reactive) in taking care of your body.

Detox/Shakes/Smoothies/Liquid Diets - Quick and Easy Food Prep

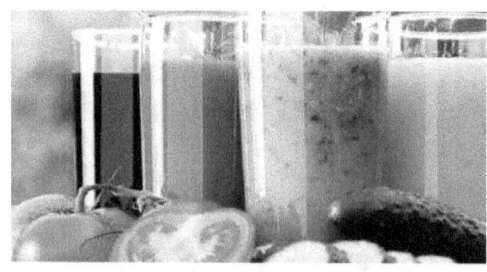

Gimmick diets, liquids or solid foods that deprive the body of a balance daily nutritional intake (including protein, carbs, fats, fiber, and foods rich in the needed vitamins and minerals for optimal body function), are not recommended for fat loss or as a lifestyle. The Internet is swarming with liquid diets, detox concoctions, fancy shakes, and smoothies promising almost instant fat loss results in just days. Some examples are the lemon cleanse, apple cider vinegar cleanse, juicing diet, 7-14-21 day cleanse programs, soup cleanse, tea detox, etc. The list is endless. Now, it's not that the food or nutrient selections in the diet program are bad, but you will not all of a sudden lose 30 pounds in 30 days *and* keep it off. Yes, you may lose some weight, but it's likely muscle, not fat. Further, the more muscle you lose, the slower your metabolism will be, the less fat you burn, and the fatter you will eventually get.

These diet methods have their place in weight loss, but are not recommended for short term total fat loss if you want to maintain a healthy, sane lifestyle. Think about it, after day 3 or 4, you may lose a few pounds but you will only gain it back later when you begin to crave real nutritional foods that fuel the body properly.

The best and most highly recommended way to cleanse the body, all while feeding the body and losing weight, is an all-natural detox program composed of fresh fruits, vegetable, meats, teas, herbs, and spices that feed the body adequately, clean out toxins, and reset your biological systems and thermostat (metabolism) to burn fat effortlessly. To get a jump start on some foods to consider in your weight loss journey, see the section on herbs, wholefoods, and superfoods.

How to Cut Calories off your Plate - Portion Size/Plates/Meals

One of the best and quickest ways to cut calories is portion control. Simply load your plate with nutrients (protein, fiber, carbs, and fats) that are high on the thermic effect list (which means it takes a lot of energy to burn), increase satiety and fullness, and are nutrient rich. They can be any variety of foods, as long as you are pulling from the right macro-nutrient categories.

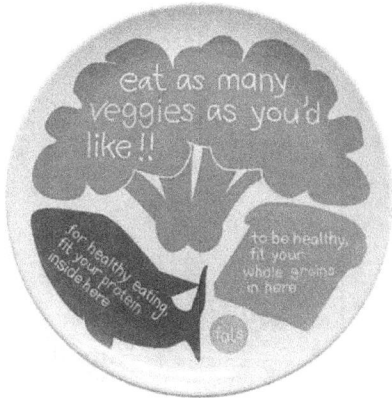

For example, a healthy plate containing 100% macro-nutrients) of 4oz wild salmon (40%), steamed broccoli (35%), and a sweet potato (20%) with coconut oil (5%) is a good illustration of a plate loaded well with adequate protein, fiber, carbs, water and fat.

As mentioned in the section on food for fuel (energy), eating protein is very filling and takes a good amount of energy to chew, breakdown, and process. By the time you get through a full chicken breast, your *"I'm full meter"* should start to kick in approximately 20 minutes from the time you start eating. Broccoli is loaded with protein, fiber, and water-based carbs. The sweet potato (approximately the size of a pear or apple) and coconut oil is a good addition to this meal for the healthy complex carbs (glucose and energy for your muscles) and essential fatty acids that provide well-balanced nutritional input.

About Vitamins, Minerals, and Supplements

The best source for essential vitamins and minerals is the foods you eat. Calcium, iron, vitamins A, B, C, D, E, and K, thiamine, niacin, magnesium, phosphorus, riboflavin, and zinc are crucial vitamins and minerals the body needs daily to function optimally and can be found readily in a variety of fruits, vegetables, meats, dairy, grains, beans, nuts, seeds, etc.

According to ACSM, people should avoid taking supplements unless specifically recommended by a physician to treat an existing nutrient deficiency disease such as low iron, vitamin D, or calcium. The use of supplements regularly tends to make individuals lazy and reduces the need to eat a quality diet high in nutrients. Most supplements are highly processed and can cause medical conditions for the user over time.

The best supplement for weight loss is to follow a high quality nutritional plan loaded with a variety of foods that include a balance of protein, fiber, carbs, water, and fat, along with adequate supplies of essential vitamins and minerals.

> *"And the best weight loss supplement is...*
> *COMMITMENT!*
> *Sold exclusively by self-determination.*
> *Visit inner-self (the mind) today and check inventory. Supplies extremely limited."*
> ~ E. Payne

Water and the Body - Why you need to drink water, daily

The human body is composed of over 60% water. According to ACSM, *"Water is needed in the body to transport nutrients to cells and carry waste away from cells. It is also serves as a lubricant for the body and through sweating, helps to maintain body temperature."*

All of our organs are composed mostly of water. Scientists suggest that the brain and heart are composed of 73% water and the lungs are about 83% water. The skin contains 64% water, muscles and kidneys are 79%, and even the bones are watery: 31%. Without water, the body will cease to function. If the body doesn't get an adequate supply of water, almost all of your major organs can be affected, especially the heart. Symptoms of dehydration will include dry mouth, thirst urgency, dry clammy skin, drop in body temperature, increased heart rate, and more. By the time you say, "I'm thirsty," your body is already down 1 to 2 liters of fluid (ACSM).

When you sweat during a workout, that's your body's cooling system, not necessarily an indication of how much fat or calories you're burning, nor is it a direct indication of how hard you're working. There are scientific formulas that can track such numbers, but understand: you can't sweat off pounds or wear plastic sweat suits hoping to lose weight faster. Why? They are designed to hold heat, causing one to sweat profusely. When wearing one during a workout, this causes your body to lose water, which could lead to dehydration, light headiness, etc.

Body weight, water weight, muscle weight, and fat weight are four different things. Body weight is the total composition of bones, tissues, fluids, and any other matter in the body. Water weight can be several things. Water weight or water retention can occur from a salty meal, following the menstrual cycle, an imbalance in body PH, kidney issues, or edema. Muscle weight or lean body mass (LBM) is the measurement of your body weight in muscle. This can be calculated using BMI, skin fold measurements, and other body composition testing (see the section "Which Weighs More: Fat or Muscle?").

Fat weight or fat mass (FM) is a measurement of your total body weight in fat. Be careful categorizing all fat mass as bad. Remember, we need fat in our bodies to survive. The goal is to keep your body fat percentage in a healthy and safe range for your age, weight, height, and body composition.

To lose weight safely and stay healthy, drink water every day -- a minimum of 64 oz. or 8 cups, to start. You'll begin to appreciate the many benefits of water beyond weight loss, such as clear, youthful skin, regular bowel movements, energy, etc.

Sugar, Salt, and Starches

Sugar is the world's most addictive, lethal, and legal drug, And, I have a confession to make -- true story about me...

I'm gonna ask that you please forgive me now for I have lived a lie for so long. I have a drug addiction I hid from my family and friends for years and I've learned that acknowledgement and confession is the first step to healing. I was introduced to these drugs at a very early age. As I grew from toddler, to teen, to young adult, the addiction became worse. I couldn't go a day without it. I had the shakes and headaches in the morning, a terrible craving during the day, and a relentless drive to get it in the evening. The signs and symptoms went unnoticed because many of my family and friends had the same issue. It wasn't until my adult years that I sought help and learned what has kept me tired, ill at times, and fighting diseases all my life.

Those drugs are SALT, SUGAR, and STARCH. Now, I know you're all probably thinking I'm crazy, but I'm not kidding. These three legalized drugs are silent killers. Yes, we need them to survive, but when they are taken in abundance they bring another entire host of issues.

On to healing...I've been in rehab for 4 years now and getting stronger each day. My rehabilitation program includes healthy eating, daily physical activity/aerobics, resistance training, and a new mindset! I've accepted my new way of life and I love it! Now, from time to time, I still get cravings for these drugs, but I have learned how to manage and limit those desires and get on to living!! Each day is a new beginning and I chose life!! If anyone can relate to what I'm saying, please join me in the race to recovery.

According to AHA, the maximum amount of added sugars you should eat in a day are: 150 calories per day (37.5 grams or 9 teaspoons) for men, and 100 calories per day (25 grams or 6 teaspoons) for women. This maximum amount is added white table sugar and should not be confused with naturally occurring sugars in fruits and vegetables or other foods. Regardless of where the sugar comes from, it will still add to your daily caloric intake (calories).

The Glycemic Index (GI) Chart - How much sugar are you eating?

One of the biggest reasons why people stay fat and get fatter is because they do not know what kinds of foods to eat. All foods, even healthy ones, are not created equal. Here's where you need to know sugar content in the foods you eat. So many times people would say to me, "I eat a lot of fruits and vegetables," not taking in to account nutrient factors like sugar/carb load that you get from eating these foods.

The Glycemic Index is one guide you can use to determine how fast your body is converting sugar/carbs to glucose. The smaller the number, the lesser the impact of sugar being absorbed quickly into the body. Using the GI chart is not a "one stop shop" for fat loss, but instead it is a tool to balance your nutritional intake. You still have to keep in mind portion size, other macronutrients eaten with carbs (protein, fats), time of day, etc.

Glycemic Index chart range
Low GI = < 60
Medium GI = 60 - 85
High GI = >85 or more

A Note on Insulin and Fat Loss

Whenever you eat any food, insulin (a hormone secreted by the pancreas) is released to stabilize the amount of sugar/glucose in the blood. Insulin has many functions in the body including facilitation of glucose getting to muscle, fat, and other tissue throughout the body to use as energy or store as fat. The body needs insulin to regulate the amount of sugar in the blood, but when there is excess sugar in the blood, insulin promotes the storage of sugar in the form of glycogen in the liver, muscles, and fat cells. This may seem like the culprit for fat gain, but the more you eat foods that continually spike your blood sugar levels (overeating), the more fat you store, furthering the onset of "insulin resistance" (when your cells stop responding to the vital role of insulin, keeping blood sugar levels down in the body). What happens when your cells stop responding? Sugar stays up and welcomes diabetes. Let's bring it home: the more high sugar/carbs/empty calorie content foods you eat (like sodas, fruit juices, cakes, pies, cookies, cracker, greasy fried foods), the more you are overeating, the higher your insulin level, the more you store body fat, the higher the likelihood of medical diagnosis (obesity, insulin resistance, diabetes, etc.).

Pass the Salt, PLEASE!

Found on every kitchen table, salt is one of the most common flavor seasonings and preservatives used in food. Salt consists of sodium chloride, is abundant in nature, and is used mostly to season or preserve food. AHA recommends *"no more than 2,300 milligrams (mgs) of salt per day and an ideal limit of no more than 1,500 mg per day for most adults."* One teaspoon of salt equals 2300 milligrams. Wow! Some of us put that on our favorite chicken and rice dish -- which doesn't include the salt already in the chicken and rice that preserves it until you eat it. I think you can see where this is leading and why you must pay attention to food labels. After looking at the sodium content on the food label, you may find it best to leave that item on the shelf.

Sea Salt or Table Salt?

The biggest differences between sea salt and table salt are how each is processed, how each tastes, and the textures of each. According to the Mayo Clinic's Katherine Zerastsky, R.D, L.D, *"Sea salt is produced through evaporation of ocean water or water from saltwater lakes, usually with little processing. Depending on the water source, this leaves behind certain trace minerals and elements. The minerals add flavor and color to sea salt, which also comes in a variety of coarseness levels. Table salt is typically mined from underground salt deposits. Table salt is more heavily processed to eliminate minerals and usually contains an additive to prevent clumping. Most table salt also has added iodine, an essential nutrient that helps maintain a healthy thyroid."*

Depending on your health goals, you can use sea salt or table salt. However, be mindful they both have about the same nutritional value and either consumed in abundance may set the stage for medical problems such as high blood pressure, heart attack, weak blood vessels, stroke, and other effects to the body biological systems. Some health alternatives to salt are Mrs. Dash, garlic, mixed herbs, and other spices seasoning (see "Herbs, Wholefoods, and Super Foods" section for more choices).

Starch - Carbs, all good or all bad?

Sugar, carbs, bread, cellulose, and glycogen are just some of the names used interchangeably with the word starch. Starches are not all bad and they do have their place in your diet. A starch is a white substance found in green plants. It is a polysaccharide or the multi-chain molecule carbohydrate found in flours, potatoes, cereals, grains, starchy vegetables, rice, pasta, cookies, crackers, etc.

Once in the body, starch is converted to glucose and later stored as glycogen in the liver and/or muscles. It becomes great fuel for energy, especially for the muscles. According to the Journal of Applied Physiology, *"Carbohydrates are the body's main energy source during high-intensity and prolonged running which means when you are engage in short burst intensity exercises, your body needs immediate fuel or energy drive these movements hence sugar is burned."*

Muscles may use carbs and fat in the body during exercise. There is a limited supply of sugar (glycogen) in the muscle for energy so when your body needs to make quick, bursting movements, sugar becomes the energy source. When walking the treadmill for one hour, walking the track, gardening, walking the mall, or other passive, subconscious movements throughout the day, the body will shift to burning fat instead. Fats have a much larger reserve for energy when the body is engaged in physical activities over a period time. At these times, fat becomes the body's go-to for energy.

Starches can be complex, like sweet potatoes, breads, grains, oats, pasta, rice, pizza, beans, etc., or simple, like certain fruits, candy, sodas, fruit juices, jellies, table sugar, syrup, etc. One difference between the two is that complex carbs take longer to breakdown in the body, whereas simple carbs are absorbed much faster into the blood stream. Both impact your blood sugar levels. No matter what kind of starch you eat and the quantity you eat, your daily movement, physical activities, and exercises will dictate how fast the starch is absorbed and used for energy, or stored as fat.

Fibrous carbs, or non-starchy water-based vegetables, are highly recommended to add to your nutrition plan. Loaded with nutrients like protein, fiber, water, and healthy carbs, these foods rank high for fat loss and a lifestyle of healthy eating because they deliver so many nutritional benefits to the body. You can eat them in large amounts, they are easy to prepare, and they taste great. Some of these foods include spinach, broccoli, kale, celery, lettuce, string beans, brussel sprouts, onions, mushrooms, zucchini (squash), cauliflower, cucumbers, and tomatoes, just to name a few.

Lastly, avoid no carb diets. They're a short term, quick fix. You may lose some weight temporarily, only to gain it back, and binge when you start eating carbs again. A no carb diet is not sustainable for a lifetime. Your body needs carbs daily to survive. It's like turbo fuel for your muscles or else you'll be a sluggish mess trying to get through the first half of the morning with no energy. I recommend a low-carb, high fiber, high protein, good fat diet because it helps you build and keep lean muscle, balance hormones, curb cravings, and burn fat effortlessly.

Alcohol, Wine, and Coffee

But what about my favorite beverages? Can I still drink them and lose weight?

One of the world's favorite pastimes is recreational drinking -- alcohol, wine, and coffee. One thing they all have in common is they taste good! Nothing wrong with foods and beverages for enjoyment. They also have high calorie content, some more than others. Now that we got the preliminaries out of the way, can I drink alcohol, wine, or coffee and still lose weight? The short answer is NO! There are many points to argue (such as some confirmed beneficial factors, especially with wine and coffee), but for the purpose of helping you reach and master your fat loss goals, we'll explore the reasons to minimize or avoid these drinks.

Alcohol, which dates as far back as a medicine for healing, is viewed today as more acceptable for enjoyment, social gatherings, celebration, relaxation, or whatever your reason for drinking it. Alcohol is a colorless and flammable liquid that is produced through the natural fermentation of sugars and yeast such as grains, molasses, starch, or sugar. It can also be produced synthetically as a by-product or by the hydration of ethylene (Webster's Dictionary). The intoxicating characteristics of wine, beer, spirits, and other drinks, are used as fuel and industrial solvent. Alcohol can have either a stimulant or depressant effect on your body. Chronic alcohol consumption causes a major shift in behavior, thinking and body movement, slurred speech, loss of coordination, irregular sensations, increased heart rate, sexual dysfunctions, birth defects, damaged liver, seizures, increase chances for diabetes, high blood pressure, stroke, and a host of circulatory, digestive, nervous, and immune system problems. Without being overly scientific here, do you see how drinking alcohol has an enormous impact on your body and fat loss? Do you see the common theme of medical issues outside of weight loss? Now, compound that with drinking alcohol and you have the perfect storm for destroying your body. If you are trying to lose the weight and get in shape for life, avoid alcohol, period! There are many other enjoyable alternatives and benefits for *not* drinking alcohol, like indulging in your favorite dessert loaded with your favorite fruit or a chocolate, vanilla or strawberry smoothie or shake, saving money (buying alcohol is an unnecessary expense), enhancing quality of life, and on and on.

Wine - "I gotta have my red wine..."

Actually, red wine is a not a bad beverage used, in moderation of course. According to the Mayo Clinic, *"Red wine, in moderation, has long been thought of as heart healthy. The alcohol and certain substances in red wine called antioxidants may help prevent coronary artery disease, the condition that leads to heart attacks. Any links between red wine and fewer heart attacks aren't completely understood. But part of the benefit might be that antioxidants may increase levels of high-density lipoprotein (HDL) cholesterol (the 'good' cholesterol) and protect against cholesterol buildup."*

While red wine might sound great with your evening meal, doctors are wary of encouraging anyone to start drinking alcohol, especially if you have a family history of alcohol abuse. Too much alcohol consumption can have harmful effects on the body. One of the huge benefits of drinking red wine is the key ingredient or antioxidant called *resveratrol*, which helps to prevent damage to blood vessels, reduces low-density lipoprotein (LDL), the bad cholesterol, and prevents blood clots (Mayo Clinic). *Resveratrol* is not an incentive to drink red wine regularly, or at all for that matter, especially if you clearly have an addiction to drinking the beverage. Most wines are made of grapes, which contain sugar even before the fermentation process, additives, etc.

The conclusion of the matter is this: do not include wine or any alcoholic beverage in your weight loss program. There are many other ways to get the same health benefits of wine in other wholefoods. Don't set yourself up for failure thinking you can handle or control your intake, or drink in moderation. Habits are hard to break, especially when you add alcohol and the chemical effects on the body to the equation.

Coffee - That cup of Joe is a must!

Starbucks, Dunkin Donuts, 7-Eleven, McDonalds, Cafe Bustelo, Columbian, Folgers, Maxwell House -- did I miss your flavor? Regular, decaf, expresso, dark, medium, light, whatever your flavor, taste, or brand, coffee seems to reign supreme as a *must have* beverage in the morning or throughout the day. Would you like half and half, whole milk, vanilla, hazelnut, or Irish cream with that?

Coffee without creamer is like a peanut butter and jelly sandwich without the peanut butter!

Beyond the fat content of creamers, sugars, and additives, coffee tastes good! One big plus is the caffeine from the coffee beans. Caffeine in coffee can vary based on the type of bean and the roasting time. According to U.S. Department of Agriculture (USDA), the average 8 oz. cup of coffee may have 95mg of caffeine. This is one of the reasons you'll find folks who exercise in the morning have a cup of Joe in their hand. According to Health Magazine, *"A Spanish study, published in the International Journal of Sport Nutrition and Exercise Metabolism, found that trained athletes who took in caffeine pre-exercise burned about 15 percent more calories for three hours post-exercise, compared to those who ingested a placebo."* If you're going to have coffee, it's recommended that you drink 1 to 2 cups day in the morning or before working out, and no more for the rest of the day.

Though coffee seems to improve endurance (exercise) and memory, lessen fatigue, and enhance overall mental functioning, too much coffee with caffeine may effect adrenal glands. According to Dr. Mercola, *"Coffee is a potent substance, and can have an adverse effect on your adrenal glands if consumed in excess."* Coffee is also a diuretic and may effect central nervous system neurotransmitters.

Should you have coffee on your weight loss journey? You don't need coffee to lose weight. If you're addicted to coffee, then the answer is "No." There are plenty of wholefood replacements to achieve the benefits of caffeine (such as teas and cocoa powder). Remember the benefit is in black coffee, not coffee loaded with your best fixings. Don't set yourself up for failure if you know drinking coffee in moderation is going to be a problem.

About your Favotite Creamer - "I gotta have my hazelnut cream, period!"

The majority of creamers on the market are not real dairy. Let's take a look at the ingredients in one.

Hazelnut Coffee Creamer by Nestle:
Water, Sugar, Partially Hydrogenated Soybean and/or Cottonseed Oil, and less than 2% of Sodium Caseinate (a Milk Derivative), Dipotassium Phosphate, Disodium Phosphate, Mono- and Diglycerides, Cellulose Gel, Cellulose Gum, Color Added, Natural and Artificial Flavors, Carrageenan

---

As you can see, most of the ingredients in this creamer are additives, chemicals put in food to preserve or improve taste. Although you don't have time to become a scientist and figure out every chemical compounds used in foods, I wanted to highlight several ingredients commonly used in foods that are clear red flags and encourage you to avoid them all together: sugar, partially hydrogenated soybean, and carrageenan.

Sugar - Any foods with added sugar should be avoided. Here is where many make the mistake in trying to lose weight: eating foods with sugar added. AHA suggests that women should have no more than 6 teaspoons of sugar, or no more than 100 calories from sugar per day. Just read the food label before eating and it will tell you how much sugar is in one serving.

Partially Hydrogenated Soybean - According to Cynthia Sass MPH, RD with SHAPE, *"A new report from the Center for Science in the Public Interest found high amounts of this unhealthy fat in numerous supermarket samples, from 4 to 5 grams per serving in microwave popcorn to a whopping 9 grams in one brand of doughnuts. With all of the media attention on sugar and salt some consumers have forgotten about trans-fat, and others mistakenly believe that it has been banned. The truth is it's still out there, and avoiding it is important for both weight control and optimal health. Partially hydrogenated oil, man-made trans-fat is created when liquid oils are made into solids, which are used to hold products like pie crust and crackers together and extend their shelf lives. Numerous studies have linked trans-fat to heart disease, infertility, cancer, type 2 diabetes, liver problems, and obesity. A weight-control study in animals found that even with the exact same number of calories and identical amounts of fat, animals fed trans-fat gained four times more weight and 30 percent more belly fat. Based on the evidence, the Dietary Guidelines for Americans state that the optimum goal for trans-fat intake is as close to zero as possible, but avoiding it can be tricky. Technically, a product can claim to provide zero grams of trans-fat if it contains less than 0.5 grams per serving. That means if it contains .4 grams and you eat 10 servings, you actually took in 4 grams, not 0. The only way to really tell if a product contains trans-fat is to check the ingredient list. If the words "partially hydrogenated" appear, bingo—there's trans-fat in the product."*

Carrageenan - According to Dr. Andrew Weil, MD, *"Carrageenan is a common food additive that is extracted from a red seaweed, Chondrus crispus, which is popularly known as Irish moss. Carrageenan, which has no nutritional value, has been used as a thickener and emulsifier to improve the texture of ice cream, yogurt, cottage cheese, soy milk, and other processed foods. Some animal studies have linked degraded forms of carrageenan (the type not used in food) to ulcerations and cancers of the gastrointestinal tract. More worrisome, undegraded carrageenan – the type that is widely used in foods – has been associated with malignancies and other stomach problems."*

Green Tea and Fat Loss

Why you should drink green tea regularly

There have been a great deal of studies and interest in green tea for boosting fat loss. The more you understand how useful certain foods can be in facilitating fat loss, the better off you'll be in attaining your goal and maintaining a healthy lifestyle.

What is green tea? It is a type of tea made from camellia sinensis leaves which originated in China and India. *"In traditional Chinese and Indian medicine, practitioners used green tea as a stimulant, a diuretic (to help rid the body of excess fluid), an astringent (to control bleeding and help heal wounds), and to improve heart health. Other traditional uses of green tea include treating gas, regulating body temperature and blood sugar, promoting digestion, and improving mental processes."* (University of Maryland Medical Center)

More studies are revealing the benefits of green tea for fat loss, and this is an important reason to consider drinking it regularly. *"Since the 1990s, green tea is also seen as a natural herb that can enhance energy expenditure and fat oxidation and thereby induce weight loss. Almost all of the studies conducted with Asian subjects have shown positive results about the anti-obesity effects of catechins. Results from study show catechins or Epigallocatechin gallate (EGCG) caffeine mixture have a small positive effect on weight loss and weight management. Studies also show a significantly decreased body weight and significantly maintained body weight after a period of time."* (International Journal of Obesity)

There are many other benefits to drinking green tea or including matcha tea and green tea extract (EGCG, epigallocatechin gallate) in your nutrition plan. They include improving immune system (green tea excellent antioxidant), boosting energy, enhancing exercise performance, and fighting cancer growth, just to name a few. Adding green tea to your daily nutrition plan can help control your appetite, enhance fat loss over time, and provide a wide variety of health benefits to keep the body performing optimally. Remember this: green tea is another tool for your weight loss arsenal but should not to be relied upon exclusively for losing weight.

Exercise

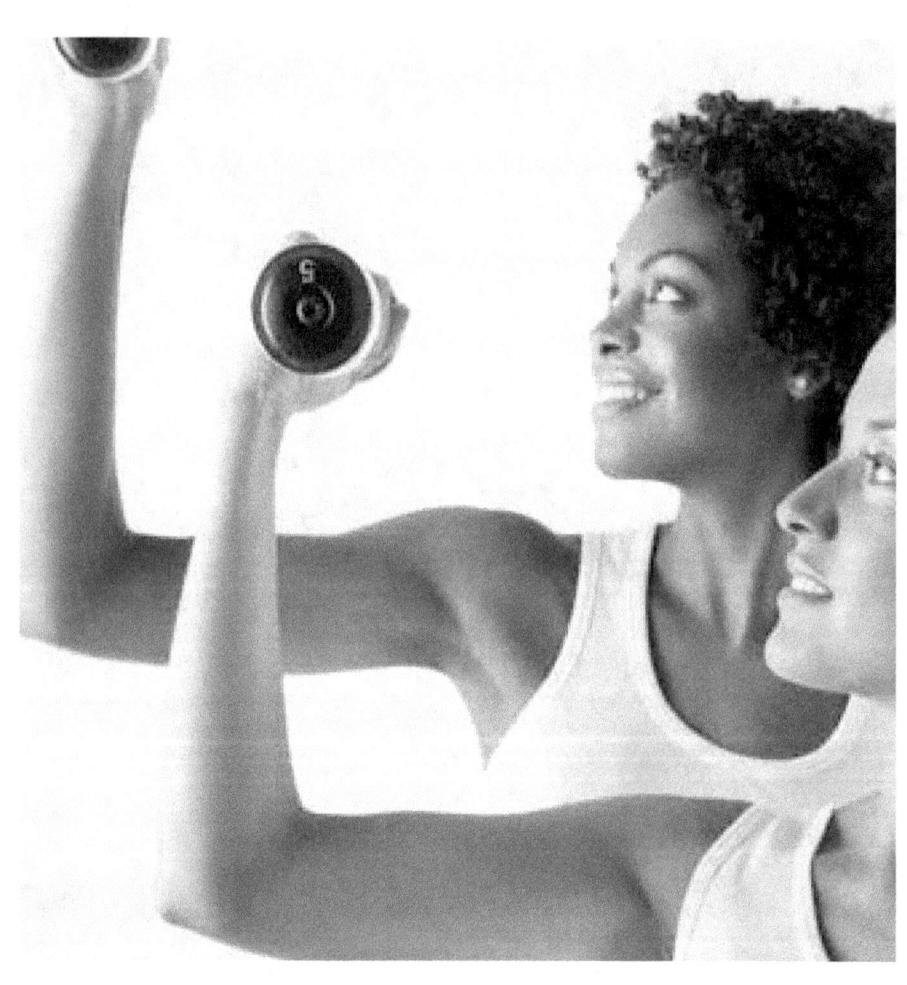

(6)

Physical activity is recommended for all age groups, men, women, and children. Our bodies are designed to move, engage, sit down, get up, and any form of movement you can think of, from sports to casual walking. Walking alone is one of the easiest, non-invasive exercises anyone can perform effortlessly, yet we live in a society where we've grown too lazy to want to move. We drive our cars one block to the store, take elevators to the first level, circle parking lots to be closest to the door, and on and on. *Use it or lose it* is the old adage, but it's true. The more you move your body, engaging different muscle groups, joints and bones, pushing pulling, lifting, standing, sitting, flexing, extending, and rotating you do, the better your body performs. Movement can decrease health issues, increase strength and endurance, improve bone density and increase energy, and rest as a means to achieving an enhanced quality of life. Who wouldn't want to chase their 5 year old grandson for 10 minutes in the park, walk the ocean front with their mate, carry groceries from market to car, walk up a flight of steps without getting winded, lift yourself out of the bed instead of rolling out, or put on your skinny jeans size 8?

The medical and health industries have a generalized standard. Unless you are engaging in physical activity on a regular basis, you are considered sedentary (which can lead to cardiovascular disease) and at risk for developing other medical problems. ACSM suggests that adults should get at least 150 minutes of moderate-intensity exercise per week, which can be met through 30 to 60 minutes of moderate-intensity exercise (five days per week) or 20 to 60 minutes of vigorous-intensity exercise (three days per week). One can do this with a brisk walk in your community, at the park, at the gym, or at the mall. To add some intensity, carry weights, walk up and down steps, walk up a hill, add some jumping jacks or stationery total body extensions to your workout. You don't need to go the gym every day. Find creative ways to engage in physical activity. Set up trips to the mall on lunch break and just walk. Not a bad view, right? You can also take mini-breaks at work walking the hallways, around the building, or to different departments, etc.

Cardio training

The most important muscle in your body is the heart. As one of the main parts of the cardiovascular system, it pumps over 1900 gallons of blood each day, and more than 50 million gallons over a 75 year lifetime (ACSM). The role of the heart is to pump blood out to the body and to receive blood coming back in from the body. Heart tissue, blood arteries, blood vessels, valves, and chambers are other components making up this vast circulatory machine that the body must have to sustain life. When any of these parts malfunction, are damaged, or die, it can compromise the entire cardiac function and other body systems.

The cardiovascular system's main purpose is to deliver nutrients to and remove metabolic waste products from tissue (ACSM). This is why cardiovascular exercise is important. It regulates efficient transportation of oxygen from heart to lungs and lungs to heart, disbursement of nutrients, balance of fluids in body, balanced PH, sustained body temperature, and removal of waste products. (ACSM).

Cardio training is great for maintaining and enhancing the cardiovascular system. These exercises including walking, running, biking, swimming, boating, hiking, and stepping, etc. The goal is to get your heart up to a sustained heart rate for approximately 30 minutes a day. Your target heart rate range for your age, gender, weight, and pulse per minute averages between 60% and 75% of your maximum heart rate. In today's market, fitness trackers like Fitbit, Apple, and Garmin are good for calculating this number for you. Incorporating cardio training into your daily routine is one of the best ways to stay active, fit, and healthy, and to burn calories effortlessly.

There are several forms of cardio training such as high intensity interval training (H.I.I.T), metabolic conditioning, aerobics classes, circuit training, or cross training all differing in time, intensity, and equipment. So you can't get bored with cardio! Deciding which form to use is literally your choice and will be determined by your body's ability to perform the exercise. Note: Performing all cardio training without some form of resistance training (weight lifting) is not recommended. Some studies suggest that strength training is better for losing belly fat than cardio. Cardio or aerobic exercise burn fat *and* muscle, but weight lifting burns fat almost exclusively. You never want to burn muscle, ever! Remember, muscle is metabolism. The more you have, the more your body burns calories at rest.

Studies also show that performing too much cardio raises cortisol (stress hormone), weakens the immune system, causes unnecessary breakdown of tissue, and disrupts sleep patterns. According to an article by Dr. Mercola, a study presented at the Canadian Cardiovascular Congress 2010 in Montreal, regular exercise reduces cardiovascular risk by a factor of 2 or 3. But the extended, vigorous exercise performed during a marathon raises cardiac risk by seven-fold! Long-distance running also leads to high levels of inflammation that may trigger cardiac events and damage your heart long after the marathon is over.

High Intensity Internal Training (H.I.I.T)

To burn calories, burn fat, and lose weight, get in shape with SMART CARDIO!

One of the more popular forms for effective fat loss is high intensity interval training (H.I.I.T), also refer to as *interval training*. This form of cardio requires you to work at near maximal heart rate, performing exercises such as squats, push-ups, sit ups, running, sprints, jump rope, running steps, etc., hence the name *high intensity*. Once you reach near maximal exertion, you slow down to lower the heart rate. The time frame for intensity can range between 10 to 30 seconds followed by a period of rest. The entire workout should last up to 30 minutes. Excess high intensity exercise over a long period of time will raise cortisol levels, stressing your body and ultimately leading to belly fat.

The reason why this form of training is highly effective for fat loss is it triggers excess post-oxygen consumption (EPOC) or after-burn effect. EPOC is the consumption of more than usual amounts of oxygen, generally increasing more after high intensity exercises than after lighter or moderate exercises (ACSM). What this means is that your body's metabolism will be higher for a longer period following this form of cardio training. Why? Because the body has to work overtime returning oxygen and other important nutrients to blood and muscle tissue all while maintaining your regular body functions. All this boils down to: *burn more calories, burn fat.* You'll do more work doing 30 minutes of H.I.I.T. than the average person walking on a treadmill for one hour. You in?

If you're more the adventurous type, cross training, cross fit, or exercises requiring a great more deal skill, stamina, strength, conditioning, and cardiovascular endurance, are other forms of cardio training you can do. The only drawback with these forms of exercise is if you're not in sports-specific shape to perform these exercises, then injuries are inevitable. *Stay in your lane.* There are plenty of alternative, safe, fun, and adventurous cardio workouts like line dancing, hiking a beginner's trail, body pump aerobics, music genre workouts, etc.

For fat loss, cardio training should not be the only physical activity in your exercise regimen. A balanced exercise program will include resistance training (weights), cardio training, and a good stretch routine.

Aerobic or Anerobic - Which one is better?

Aerobic exercise is long distance and slow pace movements like running, riding a bike, or swimming. Your body is actively using oxygen while performing aerobic exercises. Anaerobic exercise requires power, strength, and speed, such as weight lifting and sprinting which do not rely on oxygen, but instead rely on other energy sources in your muscle like glycogen (sugar). This is important to understand for fat loss so you can build a balanced exercise program using the different energy systems in the body. The more you engage the body in a variety of exercises, the harder for the body to adapt, forcing new muscle tissue, burning calories, and burning fat. Do exercises that use both energy systems, like push-ups, sit-ups, jump rope, squats, bench press, walking steps, and jogging on the treadmill for intervals. Balance is key. Performing more anaerobic exercises will trigger the after-burn effect, affording you a smarter workout in a short time frame, and allowing you to burn a lot of calories and fat while at rest.

Resistence Training, Weight Training, and Body Weight

"Because I don't wanna bulk up and look like a man..."

Fact or Myth: Women who lift weights will bulk up and look like a man.

Myth. Nothing can be further from the truth! One of the best ways to torch body fat, change your body composition, boost your metabolism, and build a lean, tone, fit body is doing resistance training. When a woman lifts weights she will not bulk up and look like a man.

One reason women can't biologically ever look like a man (without the use of steroids) is the level of testosterone she has compared to men. According to National Institute of Health (NIH), a female has 15 to 70ng/dl vs. a male who has 300 to 1,000 ng/dL (ng/dL = nanograms per deciliter). Unless a woman is taking testosterone injections or other steroids for muscle growth, she can lift weights every day and not bulk up to look like a man. There are some rare exceptions to the rule for women who may be naturally strong, carry an athletic build, or enjoy strength and conditioning training.

Here's the diamond in the rough when you lift weights:
- Stronger muscles, better performance
- Strong Core (area from abs to quads and lower back) better able to support your body weight
- Increases the number & size of calorie-torching muscle fibers
- Stronger muscles better hold your joints in position
- Trains your bones, new bone cells, bones stronger & denser (decrease susceptibility osteoporosis)
- Strength Training is Cardio!!
- Total body transformation by changing body composition
- Increase metabolism
- Improve joint mobility
- Better rest, sleep
- Better weight control

There are endless benefits to lifting weights, including weight loss. Include resistance training (weight training) in your fat loss programs and lose weight, reshape your body, and enhance your entire quality of life..

The best way to take advantage of the vast benefits of resistance training is to develop a weight lifting program targeting large muscle groups with compound exercises and movements (multiple joint movement involving more than one muscle group at a time) instead of isolated exercises focusing on one muscle group at a time. The more natural body movements you use -- with exercises working larger muscles groups first like your thighs (quads), back of thighs (hamstrings) butt (glutes) to smaller groups like chest (pecs), back (lats), shoulders, arms, abs, etc. -- the more calories you burn in one workout using all these muscles collectively.

For example, compound exercises like squats, lunges, bent row, bench press, and chin ups, to name a few, are great for burning overall body fat, building lean muscles, and reshaping your body. Isolated exercises like bicep curls, tricep extensions, or calf raises have their place in overall body sculpting and toning. If your ultimate goal is fat loss, use compound movements in your fat loss programs. As you get leaner, toner, fitter, and want to focus more on aesthetics (a certain look), isolated exercises will facilitate the look you're after by focusing on those different muscles groups.

A key concept to grasp with resistance training is incorporating components that manipulate or stress the body's cardiovascular fitness, body composition, nervous system, flexibility, and that challenge muscle groups to promote growth. ACSM suggests that beginner and advanced training options can increase the challenge of an exercise program by manipulating current exercises through the FITT-VP principle (frequency, intensity, time, type, volume and progression).

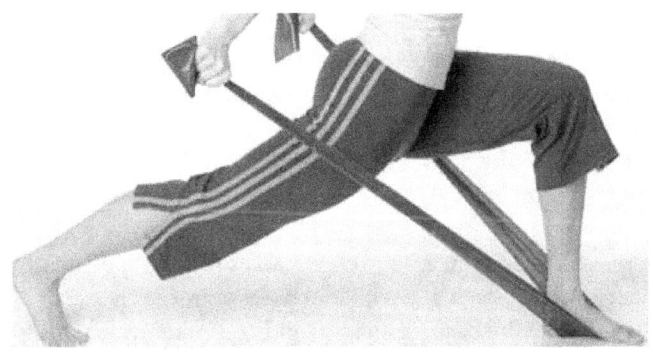

Here's what the FITT-VP principle looks like in a resistance training program:

Frequency	how often per week you lift (3-5 days a week)
Intensity	how much weight you lift and how many reps you do (this is an inverse relationship meaning the more weight you lift the fewer the reps, 8-10 repetitions for strength, growth conditioning), the less weight you lift, the more reps you can do, 10-15 repetitions for endurance
Time (duration)	how much time it take to perform set
Type (mode)	what type equipment or exercise performed (free weights, bands, body weights
Volume	how many sets you perform of exercise (3-4 sets)
Progression	increasing resistance (weight), repetitions, volume or frequency

Source: American College of Sports and Medicine (ACSM)

Overload Principle - No new challenge, No results

Go lift weights! And not only lift weights, but lift heavy weights that challenge your muscles and nervous system to build new muscle. The way you'll know whether you're growing or adapting is whether you lift the same 5 to 10 pound dumbbells weights for the last year or you graduate over a period of time to lifting 15, 20, or 25 pound dumbbells -- constantly challenge your body to grow. One way to keep lifting so the body doesn't adapt is using the *overload principle*. This principle keeps your body from adapting to the same stimulus or weight you've been lifting by adding more weight and volume (more sets) to the exercise routine. For example, if you've been lifting 10 pound dumbbells for the last couple weeks, it's time to overload by going up to 12 or 15 pounds.

This is a huge trap women fall into because we do not lift weights and when we do, we think lifting a cute, pink 5 pound dumbbell is going to bring about fat loss and a tone, fit body. Doesn't work that way. Weightlifting is one of the best ways to lose weight and tone the body, but you must lift weights and lift smart, using resistance training principles to reach your goals.

There are many other resistance training variables such as specificity of training, periodization, prioritization, variation, and others outside the scope of this book. However, if you follow the basic principles and components for using weights in your exercise programs, your fat loss results will be well worth the effort and you'll appreciate the many benefits from lifting weights.

Body Weight Exercises & Calisthenics - No gym, No track, No Equipment Needed! Just you, your body weight and that space on the side of your bed

One of the best ways to get started with resistance training is to use your own body weight. Resistance or weight training is simply you working against some type of force resisting your movement. Your body can certainly be a force to work with. When you get out of bed in the morning you have to pick yourself up (some may roll to the edge), but you're working against gravity with the use of force. Now this example is simple, but it helps you to see how walking around with your own body weight can be a workout, especially if you're overweight.

Calisthenics is gross movement without the use of equipment such as running, walking, pushing, pulling, bending, swinging, or any movement that engages large and small muscle groups. Some examples are push-ups, sit-ups, crunches, leg raises, squats, pull-ups, and lunges to name a few. Learning how to work with your own body will greatly enhance your ability to torch body fat and build a lean, tone, fit body because you force the entire body to engage a lot of muscles for each exercise.

When performing resistance training with your own body weight, your muscles have many different roles. For example, if you are doing squats, the movement requires the abs, back, and hamstrings to support or stabilize your body (synergistic muscles), while the quads and glutes (the prime movers or agonist muscles) work to perform the exercise. When you use the quads and glutes, your hamstrings, the opposing muscle or antagonist muscles are lightly engaged or relaxed. This type of movement burns a lot of calories and the best part about it, you don't need a gym. You can work at home in a small space at your own skill level and it doesn't take a lot of time to perform.

8 key principles to embrace with resistance training:
1. Lifting weights will not make you bulky or manly looking.
2. Don't wait to lose weight before lifting weights. It's the other way around. Lift weights and lose the weight at the same time while reshaping your body to a fit, lean, tone physique.
3. Resistance training, weight training, and body weight training can include cardiovascular training. Increase the intensity and volume. Get the best out of your workout.
4. Muscle is metabolism! The more muscle you have, the higher your metabolism at rest, the more total calories you burn.

5. Lift weights, lift heavy weights. Always challenge your body with new stimuli (weight). Aim for a quality workout.
6. You don't need gym membership to lose weight. You need to commit to your fat loss journey. Work with the matter between your two ears first and the rest will follow.
7. Muscle will not turn into fat nor will fat turn into muscle. They are two different tissues. You can lose muscle (bad) and gain fat (worse). Instead, build and keep lean muscle and lose fat effortlessly.
8. Women can and should lift weights. The more you challenge your body with resistance training, the more you'll boost fat loss, drastically reshape your body, and enhance your biological systems tremendously, all while building a lean tone, fit, and healthy body regardless of your age.

Spot Reduction - "I wanna pick and choose where on my body to lose weight..."

Most women generally want to perform exercises targeting certain areas on the body while trying to preserve others. This is known as spot reduction. This term has evolved as one of the biggest market tools used by gyms, trainers, equipment producers, and fad exercise craze gurus.

It does not work. You can't tell the body (your genetic code) how and where you want to lose weight. Weight loss is distributed physically according to your genetics. Now, this doesn't mean that hard work on specific body parts like your abs -- doing 1000 crunches, sit-ups, and side bends -- won't net some kind of change. At best, you'll get tired, sore, or injured, with a bigger, harder belly, and frustrated you're not seeing any results. *"Spot reduction doesn't burn a lot of calories and they don't help in a major way with fat loss,"* says Wayne Westcott, PhD, professor of exercise science at Quincy College in Quincy, Massachusetts. Crunches are not the answer to flat abs -- instead, the best approach to overall fat loss is a balanced nutrition and exercise program, and reduced stress (cortisol levels).

Can't Out-Train a Bad Diet - "I can work it off later..."

Here's another myth that keeps individuals in the dark: **You can out train a bad diet -- as long as you are working out you can eat what you want.** Wrong! You can't eat what you want and think you're going to work it off later. I tried it for years only to get frustrated -- until I started doing it the right way by developing a lifestyle of good nutrition and exercise.

Consider the following scenario:

Average calories burned/hour: Aerobic exercise 457 calories, 155lb person

Average Daily Caloric Intake requirements: Between 1700-2100 calories

Average Meal: 400-650 calories

Do you see why you can't work off what you just ate? You can literally wipe out your calories burned in an hour workout with one snack. Avoid the trap of thinking you can eat what you want when you want to, especially if you are trying to lose weight. Now, this doesn't include an occasional indulgence in your favorite foods from time to time. But if you have a loose nutritional program, eating with no concern about what you're putting in your mouth, then working out that evening or the next morning thinking, *"This workout is for yesterday's greed..."* you will be disappointed when you notice you're getting fatter, your cravings increase, and you're not reaching any of your fitness goals. At the end of the day fat loss and a sustained healthy lifestyle is approximately 80% nutrition and 20% exercises.

Eat Best, Exercise Smart

"Should I eat less and exercise more or eat more and exercise less?"

The immediate thought process for most women is to walk the treadmill or track, or to do aerobics seven days a week, and eat like a bird nibbling on fruit, salads, and water. Stop! Starving yourself to death and jumping into every aerobics class you can find is not the way to lose weight effectively and keep it off.

We have to change our thinking and understand what *metabolism* is and how it works. Metabolism is a life sustaining chemical process in the body that converts the foods you eat to energy, and provides the body what it needs to function. When you decide to starve the body of fuel (energy) and workout excessively, the body will seek to compensate for the loss of energy (food) by slowing down your metabolism, using your muscle as energy (breaking down protein), therefore causing you to lose muscle and store body fat. Metabolism can also have an opposite effect: if you exercise more and smarter (using fat torching exercises and movement), while eating more of the right food, you can build lean muscle tissue all while burning fat.

Dr. Teta, in "Metabolic Effect," suggests --

> "...The first step to beating stubborn fat is to stop dieting. Eating less, and exercising more activates alpha receptors and suppresses beta receptors if taken to the extreme. This is because stress can cause issues with insulin and thyroid among other hormones that alter physiology in favor of alpha receptors over betas. As a reminder, beta receptors are like big garage doors that let fat out quickly (B for beta and burn). Alphas are like tiny little windows that let fat out only slowly. As my father would say, "it's like trying to put a marshmallow in a piggy bank" (A for alpha and anti-burn). Since dieting can push things in an unfavorable direction you want to take another approach. You do this by moving from an eat less, exercise more approach to either an eat less, exercise less (ELEL) or eat more, exercise more (EMEM) approach."

Balance is key here and you have to build a balanced diet high in protein, fiber, water, and healthy fats, along with fat torching compound movements and the resistance training that works best for your body.

Responsibility and Accountability

Should I hire a personal trainer? Join a gym? Buy a treadmill?

One of the biggest challenges to weight loss is the mind. Let me define this further here. We think in order to lose weight, we need to hire, buy, rent, or lease the best people, places, and things to get results. Not so. The idea of weight loss, fat loss, being fit, and healthy, etc. all starts in the mind. You have to make the commitment! See, if you have not counted the cost of what it takes to achieve your fat loss goals and the time, energy, and tools required to help you along the way, you will fail every time, just like I did.

It's not the external factors that get results, but sound beliefs systems and core values, the right spiritual fortitude (mental commitment), and having faith in yourself to achieve your personal health goals in spite of the odds. Go back and read chapter 1, then change your thinking. Romans 12:1-2 says it best, *"I beseech you therefore, brethren, by the mercies of God, that ye present your bodies a living sacrifice, holy, acceptable unto God, which is your reasonable service. And be not conformed to this world: but be ye transformed by the renewing of your mind, that ye may prove what is that good, and acceptable, and perfect, will of God."*

Get your head in the game first, before you go spend any time or money on outside resources.

Once you've commited to yourself (personal goals), then you'll be ready to build your team of influence -- which may include hiring a personal trainer (because you know you're not going to workout unless someone holds you accountable), or purchasing some dumbbells, a treadmill, or a Stairmaster to use in your home (because you know you'll commit at least 60 minutes a day to the resistance and cardio or you need to feel like you're going to the gym to workout). Any of these modes to get you going are fine as long as they work for you and you've committed physically and spiritually to using the tools and resources to lose weight and stay fit for life.

The case for the Personal Trainer

While I was on my fat loss journey, consuming a proper diet and exercising, I began to realize I could only go so far on what I knew. Even further, my results varied and I grew frustrated and stopped going to the gym. A friend recommended a personal trainer and I didn't think it would matter, but I was wrong. Not only did my trainer help me lose over 70 pounds of body fat, but I kept if off and grew passionate about helping other women reach their physical and spiritual potential to drop the weight, stay in shape, and make it a lifestyle.

Before you hire a personal trainer -- and not just any trainer -- you want to know if he or she knows about women's fat loss and has had success with their program. ACSM suggests that your trainer should not only know the basics for fat loss, but he or she should have a good understanding of the following:
- Anatomy and physiology
- General nutrition
- Kinesiology (study exercise and movement in daily living)
- Biomechanics (study of motion and the cause)
- Exercise physiology (how the body responds and adapts to exercise)
- Fitness assessment (how to conduct one accurately to build the right program)
- Expertise at applying what they know
- Common sense (knowing everybody will not *fit* into the same exercise program or mold, and building the nutrition and exercise program around the individual and not the other way around)

Above all, what has the personal trainer done to successfully helped someone to lose weight? Ask the personal trainer for testimonials, success stories, and real people that participated in their program and had fat loss success. At the end of the day, you want to lose the weight. If a personal trainer gives an exercise prescription and doesn't guarantee fat loss results or your money back, be very careful about proceeding with him or her.

Hiring a personal trainer is not too different from calling your medical doctor to take care of a problem you don't know how to fix, and he or she is the specialist or expert. For years, personal trainers have been viewed as a luxury or for people that had money to afford private training. In today's society, it's a necessity more than ever. With 1/3 of the U.S. population categorized as obese, it's an epidemic and we are in dire need of a doctor!

According to The Bureau of Labor Statistics, *"Employment of fitness trainers and instructors is projected to grow 8 percent from 2014 to 2024, about as fast as the average for all occupations. As businesses, government, and insurance organizations continue to recognize the benefits of health and fitness programs for their employees, incentives to join gyms or other types of health clubs are expected to increase the need for fitness trainers and instructors."*

It's your choice. I can't tell you whether you should hire a trainer or not; I can only share from personal experience how helpful it could be to add this tool to your fat loss journey. Unlock your brain from "I can't afford it," and set your heart on the value of your life. You can't afford not to do anything if you are diagnosed as obese and headed for hypertension, diabetes, cholesterol, or a host of other deadly diseases. I am painting the picture of gloom and doom because we have replaced our values and beliefs with the lies that we've told ourselves over the years. We're stuck there, and we won't move. What is it going to take for you to see that you are sick? Self-diagnosis, pills, and household remedies haven't cut the weight. Actually, every year the doctor tells you you're getting fatter, older, and more at risk for major medical issues. This is a true definition of *insanity*, doing the same thing and expectng different results.

I've learned over the years that when you really want something badly, you either find a way or find an excuse. Which one will you do? Are you a *way maker* or do you make excuses? Careful how you answer this very personal question, for if you look at your decision-making in other aspects of your life, you'll clearly see which one fits you well. Let's take for example, that trip to Costa Rica you plan every year and pay on it monthly until its paid for, or your bi-weekly appointment to the salon for a hairstyle, pedicure, and manicure, or that lavish full course meal at your favorite restaurant you pay for while gulping down thousands of calories in one hour. See my point? We have full control, ability, and money to spend on things dear to our hearts, things we value, cherish, and we'll do it again and again. *Do you value your health?*

Lifestyle

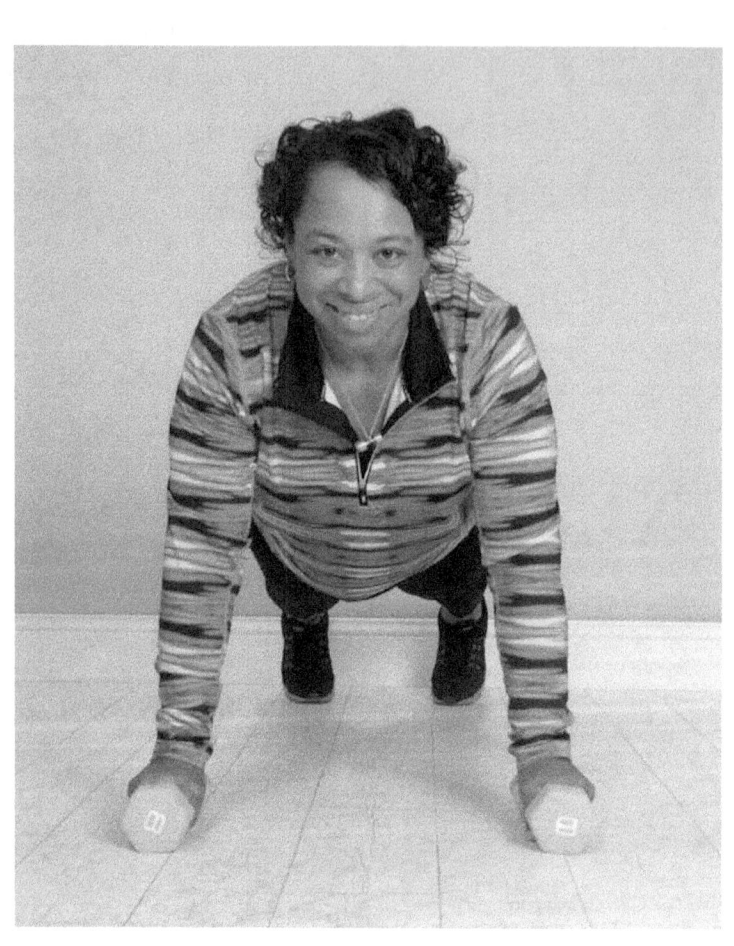

(7)

Fit, Fabulous, Fortified, and Free for Life!

"So how do I drop the weight and stay in shape and get fit for life?"

All the key concepts you've read up to this point -- from getting your mind right for your fat loss journey, to understanding the female body, choosing the right foods for your diet and nutrition program, to smart exercise and movement -- have laid the foundation for developing and maintaining a lifestyle of healthy eating and exercise. No *one concept* should be used exclusively to lose weight. The real challenge is knowing what to do and how to do it -- but you must put to work all you've learned.

So, what is *lifestyle*? Webster's dictionary defines lifestyle as a typical way of living, behaviors associated with, reflecting or promoting a desirable or particular way of living. When you use the concepts for fat loss, they become almost second nature. You'll do them regularly without hesitation or an excuse why you can't. For example, preparing your meals for the next work week will become a priority. You'll spend a few hours on the weekend at the market, herb store, or farmers market picking up your nutritional requirements for the week. Even if you don't have time to prepare meals for every day, you know where to pick up nutritional breakfast or lunch foods like mixed greens, nuts, organic meats or smoothies and shakes loaded with protein, fiber, and healthy fats. You'll make no excuses because you already know you're not eating at McDonald's, TGI Fridays, or Subway for a quick meal. Instead you visit Whole Foods, Trader Joe's, or the next best quick yet healthy nutritional meal you can buy and eat in 30 minutes and get on back to work. As the saying goes, "If you fail to plan, you plan to fail." Don't get caught without a strategy for what you're going to eat, or when you're going to eat it -- which is very important to your metabolism.

Depending on your nutrition plan and exercises program, you may schedule yourself to eat 5 to 6 meals (3 full meals and 2 to 3 snacks) spaced out over three hour increments. Some prefer 3 square meals a day. I highly recommend the first because it keeps your fueled (energized) throughout the day, not too full, not too hungry because it keeps your metabolism humming along with adequate energy to perform exercises and daily movement. There are some instances where I switch to 3 meals a day. These are on days when my movement and energy expenditure is low. I don't exercise on these days; instead, I concentrate on relaxation, recovery, lowering my stress levels and gradual movement. A stroll in the park or around the mall is the most active I am on these days. The less energy (calories) you put out the less you have to take in. Or else you'll overeat if you eat the same or more on days you don't need additional food.

Overeating leads to weight gain. Remember, it becomes a necessity to eat the foods that nourish your body. If you go a meal without them, you'll get immediate feedback from your body in the form of a headache, cravings, sluggish feeling, decreased mental sharpness, loss of energy, and in most instances, guilt because you know you didn't eat the right best foods for your body. Find the balance and strategies that work for your life and feel free to switch between them, knowing ang planning for the activity (exercises) and nutrition.

Other lifestyle habits to develop are not eating after 8pm, eating 3 hours before going to bed, or eating only within in a certain time frame (also known as intermittent fasting). Everybody fasts at some point, which is generally when you go to sleep. The goal is to get 8 to 12 hours of fasting from the time you go to sleep to the time you wake up -- no food. Then you "break the fast," or have breakfast.

Each strategy has its own benefits unique to your goals, but for the best fat loss results, naturally and effortlessly, allow your body to take full advantage of 8 to 12 hours of fasting while you sleep. Then you eat within a given time frame, which encourages fat loss.

According to Dr. Mercola, *"Intermittent fasting is a type of scheduled eating plan where you adjust your normal daily eating period to an hours-long window of time without cutting calories. Intermittent fasting is a powerful approach to eating that is becoming very popular because it can help you lose weight without feeling hunger, and help reduce your risk of chronic diseases like diabetes and heart disease. If done correctly, intermittent fasting can also lead to better sleep and lots of energy."*

Today, modern science has proven that fasting yields the following benefits:
1. Helps promote insulin sensitivity – Optimal insulin sensitivity is crucial for your health, as insulin resistance or poor insulin sensitivity contributes to nearly all chronic diseases
2. Normalizes ghrelin levels, also known as your "hunger hormone"
3. Increases the rate of hGH production, which has an important role in health, fitness, and slowing the aging process
4. Lowers triglyceride levels
5. Helps suppress inflammation and fight free radical damage

*Notes and reference from Dr Mercola,
"Everything You Need to Know about Intermittent Fasting"

Go Workout!

Keep your fitness appointments with yourself

One of the most important decisions you'll make for your lifestyle is when to work out. The haphazard attitude, "I don't have time to exercise," is probably one of the worst lies you can tell yourself. We find time to do the things we want to do. You may not want to exercise sometimes, or not at all, but it's a need for your entire physical, mental, and spiritual well-being. Exercise has been proven to fight against diabetes, high blood pressure, cholesterol, obesity, cancer, and a host of other medical diseases. According to the Centers for Disease Control and Prevention (CDC), physical activity can help control weight, reduce cardiovascular disease and the risk of some cancers, type 2 diabetes, and metabolic syndrome, strengthen bones and muscles, improve mental health and mood, prevent falls, improve ability to do activities, and increase your chances to live longer.

Finding the place, time, and type of exercise is entirely up to you. But you gotta do it. No excuses. Just like we find the time to go to the mall and shop, go to the movies, buy your favorite pair of shoes, or take a trip to the Caribbean, find time to take care of your body, your God-given temple. Make it a priority. According to ACSM, all healthy adults aged 18 to 65 years should participate in moderate intensity, aerobic physical activity for a minimum of 30 minutes on 5 days per week, or 20 minutes per day for 3 days of vigorous intensity aerobic activity. Physical activity such as walking, jogging, riding a bike, aerobic classes, lifting weights, and sports are just some options. Find an activity you enjoy for 30 minutes a day and do it! Invite family, friends, or coworkers to join you. You'll be saving your life and helping someone else too. Also, 2 is better than 1 and it can help push you through your workout.

Get your calendar out, plan at least 3 to 5 days a week that you'll go to the gym, and keep the appointment. It's that simple. If you have to cancel, reschedule, move the time up or back, do it, but keep your "health and wellness date" all the time. Let's do it!

Shake it Up!

Who wants a milkshake?

Well, not exactly. But you sure can create many tasty ways to enjoy a healthy whey protein smoothie or protein shake to help with building lean muscle tissue, appetite control, weight management, strengthening immune system, and boosting cardiovascular system. Whey protein (which comes from cows milk) is one of the best sources of high quality protein and is digested quickly in the body. You can purchase it in powder form and different flavors. There are many distributers of whey protein, so to make sure you're getting a quality whey protein powder, look for whey that delivers a balance of amino acids (both essential and nonessential, especially branch chain amino acids or BCAAs, leucine, isoleucine, and valinie), is high in protein (at least 20 to 25 grams per serving), and is low in carbs and sugar additives. According to the Journal of the American College of Nutrition, compared to soy, whey protein is higher in leucine, is absorbed more quickly and results in a more pronounced increase in muscle protein synthesis.

There is also another derivative from cow's milk called casein or *curds*. Casein is composed of about 80% milk protein and absorbs more slowly than whey. Depending on your workout schedule and lifestyle, consuming casein versus whey is not a huge choice to make, other than satiety or how quickly you need nutrients to be absorbed.

A note on soy: There have been a great deal of studies and hype about whether to eat soy and its negative impacts on health. Let's take a look. Soy, which comes from soybean plants, is another source of protein found in soy milk, soy cheese, soybean oil, soy burgers, soy ice cream, soy nuts, soy sauce, tofu, tempeh, and a host of other plant base foods with soybeans as the base. Soy is high in protein, fiber, omega-3 and a number of other healthy nutrients. Some studies show soy can help fight heart issues, cancer, loss of bone, and improve the immune system. More recent studies have shown some evidence that consuming too much soy can age brain cells causing cognitive dysfunction, digestive issues, impair thyroid, cancer, heart issues and an increase estrogen levels in men and women. For men, one known effect is enlarged breasts or "man boobs." In women, an increase in estrogen can wreak havoc on hormonal balance, and cause weight gain and stubborn fat pockets (especially around the hips, butt and thighs). According to the Journal of Nutrition, "*The interest in hormonal effects of soy in premenopausal women has centered mainly on the potential benefits of antiestrogenic effects on estrogen-dependent cancers such as breast cancer. here has been some concern that consumption of phytoestrogens might exert adverse effects on men's fertility, such as lowered testosterone levels and semen quality.*" The marginal outcomes of studies show that there should be some degree of concern and awareness about eating soy regularly in your diet.

The biggest thing to remember with food consumption, in this case soy, is what the benefits are. If you can find other foods where you can get at least the same nutritional and health benefits and limit your body exposure to health issues, then go with the better food choice. Less than 5% of my diet includes soy products. This is because I choose foods that are better and have the same nutritional benefits as soy, thereby avoiding potential negative impacts of eating soy products. Some of those foods are quinoa, whey protein, organic meats, beans, and legumes not derived from soybean. Instead of soy milk, I drink 100% unsweetened almond milk or rice milk. There are always alternatives.

Living a Balanced Lifestyle and Getting your Rest

Everything doesn't have to be perfect, but learning how to balance lifestyle is key.

There is nothing more important to me than getting my rest, all of it! Sleep, rest, stress, hormones, diet, exercise, family, children, friends, work, school, church, community, society, etc. -- there is so much to balance in life so in order to keep you healthy and in a position to help someone else, you first have to learn how to balance your own plate.

The body needs to get a fair amount of rest daily to replenish, rejuvenate, and prepare for the next 24 hours. Think about it. You spend an average of 16 hours or more per day awake, moving around, working, etc. The other 8 hours should be spent asleep, but because of stress and the many loads we take on in our personal lives (work, deadlines, etc.), the average person may only get up to 4 to 6 hours of broken sleep making it difficult to perform daily tasks and responsibilities. Not good. According to the National Sleep Foundation, adults (26 to 64 years) should be getting 7 to 9 hours of sleep every night.

When the body doesn't get proper rest, not only will your fat loss progress slow to a halt, but many biological systems in the body will be negatively effected and the environment in the body will be prime for diseases. According to the American Journal of Epidemiology, women who reported sleeping 5 or fewer hours per night were at greater risk for weight gain and in general weighed more compared with women who slept 7 to 8 hours per night.

Another research study conducted by the American Academy of Sleep Medicine Sleep Research Society suggested that *"sleep deprivation contributes to a number of molecular, immune, and neural changes that play a role in disease development, independent of primary sleep disorders. These changes in biological processes in response to chronic sleep deficiency may serve as etiological factors for the development and exacerbation of cardiovascular and metabolic diseases and, ultimately, a shortened lifespan. Sleep deprivation also results in significant impairments in cognitive and motor performance which increase the risk of motor vehicle crashes and work-related injuries and fatal accidents."*

Stop stressing, go to bed at night, and make it a priority to get your rest. You are your best investment and asset. Live in a way that demonstrates that by getting 7 to 9 hours of sleep every night. You may even dial back the clock on your age.

The Danger Zone

Avoid foods that wreak havoc on your hormones, cause inflammation, keep you fat, sluggish, out of shape, and on the express way to medical issues. There are some foods you automatically know you should avoid! Fried foods, heavily processed meats, fruits, vegetables (sold at fast food restaurants), wheat/grain products, gluten, soy, most dairy products (except eggs), white sugar, crackers, cookies, and cakes, just to name a few. Sounds like the entire food market, right? Not exactly. The reason why these particular foods are in the danger zone is because they disrupt or damage the metabolic process, create a toxic environment in the body, increase internal inflammation, cause immediate storage of body fat (most of these foods have no nutritional value), affect your major biological systems, and cause a host of chronic medical issues (obesity, diabetes, high blood pressure, cholesterol, etc.).

If you've been regularly eating these foods for years, you are creating the perfect storm for metabolic shut down or, in laymen terms, a medical disease on the rise. Your daily nutrition should not be laden with these foods, because if they are, you must change your lifestyle and approach to food choice immediately and replace your daily diet with at least 80% of clean eating. Yes! Fresh fruits, veggies, organic meats, healthy shakes, etc. Remember, the goal is to establish a lifestyle of regularly eating healthier foods. You start by removing bad foods from your diet and replacing them with healthier choices. For example, if you eat french fries, white potatoes, bread, biscuits, etc. every day, replace this entire food group with either brown rice, sweet potato, quinoa, or ezekiel bread. Small changes over time will help you develop healthier habits you will do naturally. Stop torturing your body by putting junk in it and work at feeding your body foods loaded with vitamins, minerals, nutrients, and energy!

The process of getting rid of junk foods and replacing them with healthier choices took me years to master. I had to feed and conditioned my body to crave healthy foods. Yes! When your hormones are functioning properly and your metabolism is in sync, your body will desire nothing but the best in fruits, veggies, choice meats, water, and foods that provide a great source of nutrition. I still eat the things I love, like occasionally having cake, pie, and ice cream if I desire, but these instances are very rare, sometimes on occasions like vacation or a planned dinner outing. Find your balance, experiment with different foods, taste, texture, satiety, nutrition, and enjoy good eating.

Grains, Wheat and Gluten

Why grains, wheat, and gluten should not be a part of your regular nutrition plan

You're probably wondering, *What do grains, wheat and gluten foods have to do with fat loss and lifestyle?* In previous chapters, we discussed the effects of inflammation on your system and the damage it can cause to your body. Grains, wheat, and foods with gluten can cause inflammation. Gluten is a protein found in grains, and most diets or nutrition plans include grains. All grains aren't created equal and all grains are not good for your body -- this is why it's important to create a lifestyle of understanding the foods you eat. According to the Nutrition Journal, recent animal and cell-culture models have found that elements in gluten can stimulate inflammation. While these findings are far from conclusive and require human correlation, they do conjure intriguing speculation given the current gluten-free dietary trend. Though oatmeal is at the top of the list for healthy breakfast foods, it is a grain and does contain some gluten. You don't need to ban oatmeal from your diet. But if you have allergies to gluten, be sure to find out how the oats you consume are manufactured and processed.

Eat Quinoa Instead

This super food can be eaten breakfast, lunch or dinner!

Though classified as a grain, quinoa does not have the same negative effects of wheat or gluten. Quinoa, from the leafy green vegetables family, is a pseudo-grain high in protein, fiber, magnesium, and copper, supplying all nine essential amino acids (nutrients the body can't produce on its own). It is a gluten-free food loaded with health benefits like boosting immunity (high in antioxidants), lowering blood sugar levels, and aiding the digestive system (high in fiber). It is a good source of omega-3s (healthy fat), prevents cancer, fights a host of diseases, and ultimately helps with weight loss. It also comes in different varieties and can be eaten hot or cold.

According to the Harvard School of Public Health, eating a bowl of quinoa a day may lower your risk for premature death from diseases like cancer, heart disease, respiratory disease, and diabetes by 17 percent. Best of all, it tastes great! Eat up and enjoy quinoa in salads, side dish to meats, for breakfast instead of oatmeal, in place of breads, rice, and other carbs.

Tips for Breaking Plateaus

Gotta switch up the rhythm

"I have 15-20 pounds of stubborn body fat that won't come off." I hear this a lot from individuals who've lost a lot of weight only to get inches from their ideal safe and healthy weight and can't seem to torch that last bit of body fat. Welcome to the plateau, where your body has adapted to your regular eating, exercise and lifestyle moments. You're in balance! That's great if you want to maintain that weight, but not good if you still have more to lose.

A plateau by definition is a state of no change after a time of activity or progress. Plateaus are common with fat loss progression and you'll have to break them more than once. Your body will always seek balance, meaning as you lose weight, get leaner, tighter, healthier, and more fit, after a time your body will work to maintain that metabolic state by taking in and releasing energy to keep in balance. Plateaus can be related to how you think or approach your fat loss journey, exercise type and intensity (cardio, weight training), diet or daily nutritional plan, medical issues, stress, or a combination of all of these.

Here's how you break a plateau:
Evaluate your fat loss journey after each major break point, such as after losing 10 pounds in 6 weeks, dropping 2 inches a month, or having worked out for 2 months with no change. Go back and read the sections in this book on cardio resistance training, diet, nutrition, and movement. You will need to make changes in your routine to get new results. You also need to evaluate your attitude. Ask yourself, *"Am I giving it all I've got, or am I doing just enough to get by?"* Your attitude about and perception of how hard you are working on your weight loss program, as well as your attitude about nutrition, can be huge at cracking the plateau and getting the scale moving again. Maintain a positive, honest attitude with yourself and make changes where you can. Other ways to break a plateau include increasing your resistance training, intensity, and volume, incorporating different exercises, increasing or decreasing cardio training, and switching food choices (macronutrients). You can also eat more nutritious foods, eat less than normal but more quality foods, take a break, relax, or count calories. I do not advocate the latter unless you are detailed and willing to track everything you eat and log it daily, otherwise it won't work. Breaking plateaus is simply making a change to your routine and tracking the results. After 4 to 6 weeks of a new fat loss program, you should notice some differences in pounds, inches, new muscle growth, etc. If not, there is something you're not addressing and you need to go back and re-evaluate. Don't be afraid to do this because it's normal. Just be patient and put forth your best efforts in all areas to bring about new results.

For the Traveler Always on the Go

"I don't have time to cook or go to the gym"

Developing a lifestyle of healthy eating, exercise, and living in balance is all about smart planning, better food choices, and incorporating your health and wellness as a way of life no matter where you are, on travel, or with changes in jobs, pay, people, places or things. It simply becomes a part of you, naturally. Therefore, if you have a job or lifestyle that requires you to be on the go all the time, then planning is a must!

Before you head to your destination, you should have already mapped out your health and wellness plan -- when and where you'll to eat, what you're going to eat, when you'll work out (whether in gym or in hotel room), and when you'll get your rest. No exceptions!

Here's what you do. If you regularly eat fruits, veggies, fresh organic meats, shakes, salads, nuts, etc., then you get on the Internet, get a phone book or tap in to the local healthy wholefoods restaurants, and find out who sells what you eat. They are everywhere, you just have to take time and find them. All you need is access to buy meals prepared similar to how you eat at home. An Internet search of farmers markets, wholefood markets, and healthy restaurants is a great way to find your food. And don't be afraid to ask them how it is prepared. Worst case on the go, you can always pop in to a food mart and get a bag of almonds (unsalted), healthy low sugar shake, or a piece of fruit to hold you over until you have a real meal. Lastly, you can carry a couple of whey protein powder packs, a container and some water for a quick meal.

Do you see my point? There is no reason why you can't keep your lifestyle on the road unless you don't want to. Stop telling yourself lies like, *"I couldn't find any places to eat."* That's definitely an excuse!

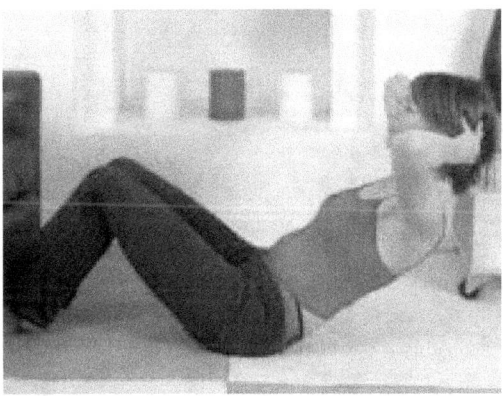

Conclusion of the Matter

(8)

Set Your Heart - COMMITMENT

"For where your treasure is, there will your heart be also." Matthew 6:21

When I thought about writing this book, my goal was to give women insight on how to drop the weight, get in shape, and live a fit, fabulous, fortified, and free life in Christ. There is so much more I can say, but I hope enough was said to get you thinking and moving.

The most important concept in this book is understanding the physical and spiritual connection, first. Until you get a strong, clear reason *why* you need to lose weight, get in shape, or take better care of your body, any avenue you try will last only a short while before you relapse and go back to your old ways.

You have to change your thinking. *Deprogram* lies, old belief systems, negative thoughts and ways, and in some instances, ignorance, and *reprogram* your thinking with truth, positive energy, spiritual discernment, and balance to choose what's right, better, and best (Romans 12:1-2). Stop choosing to be ignorant, lazy, or neglectful, and embrace power, love, and a sound mind in the body of Christ (2 Timothy 1:7).

"Wherefore be ye not unwise, but understanding what the will of the Lord is." Ephesians 5:17.

Be proactive at getting a better understanding of your God-given purpose and take the best care of your God-given temple because you represent Christ. Strive to make every effort to present your best before the Lord and the world. And then keep on praying, studying, learning and living in a way that exemplifies the love of Christ for you and all you connect with (James 1:5, Matthew 27:36-40).

The first place to start is with a self examination. Questions like:
- What do I value?
- What's important to me? Do I really care about my health or not?
- What would Jesus say or do if we were having a conversation about my health?
- Am I "…a living sacrifice, holy, acceptable unto God, which is my reasonable service?"
- What kind of example am I to my mate, children, family, friends, community, andthe Kingdom of God?
- Do I want to get better, or get worse and burden my family?
- Do I really believe my quality of life will change for the better?

- Who do I need to include in my circle to help me succeed?
- What will it cost financially? Emotionally?
- Am I ready to commit to myself and keep that commitment?

Ask yourself these questions and many more. Whatever it takes, make the sacrifice and take care of your body.

I pray that this book, if nothing else, helps you to change at least one wrong perspective you had about fat loss and replace it with truth and action to get results.

The day you fully embrace the spiritual mindset first and understand your purpose and God's plan for your life, then you'll connect the dots -- between your physical fitness and all the tools and resources outlined in this book so you can start your fat loss journey to living a *Fit, Fabulous, Fortified, & Free* life in the Lord!"

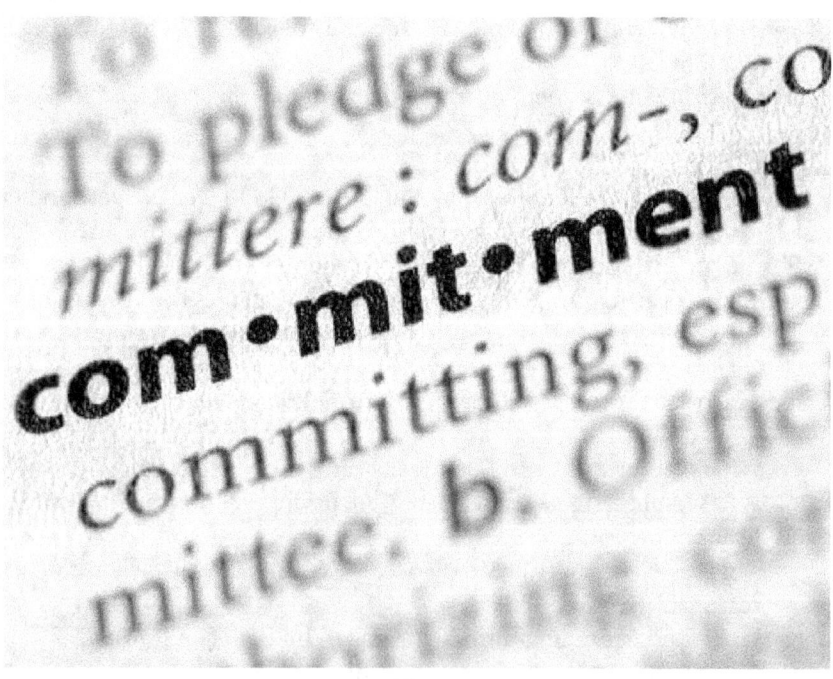

Ericka

Blasted off 70 pounds of body fat!

Before...

After...

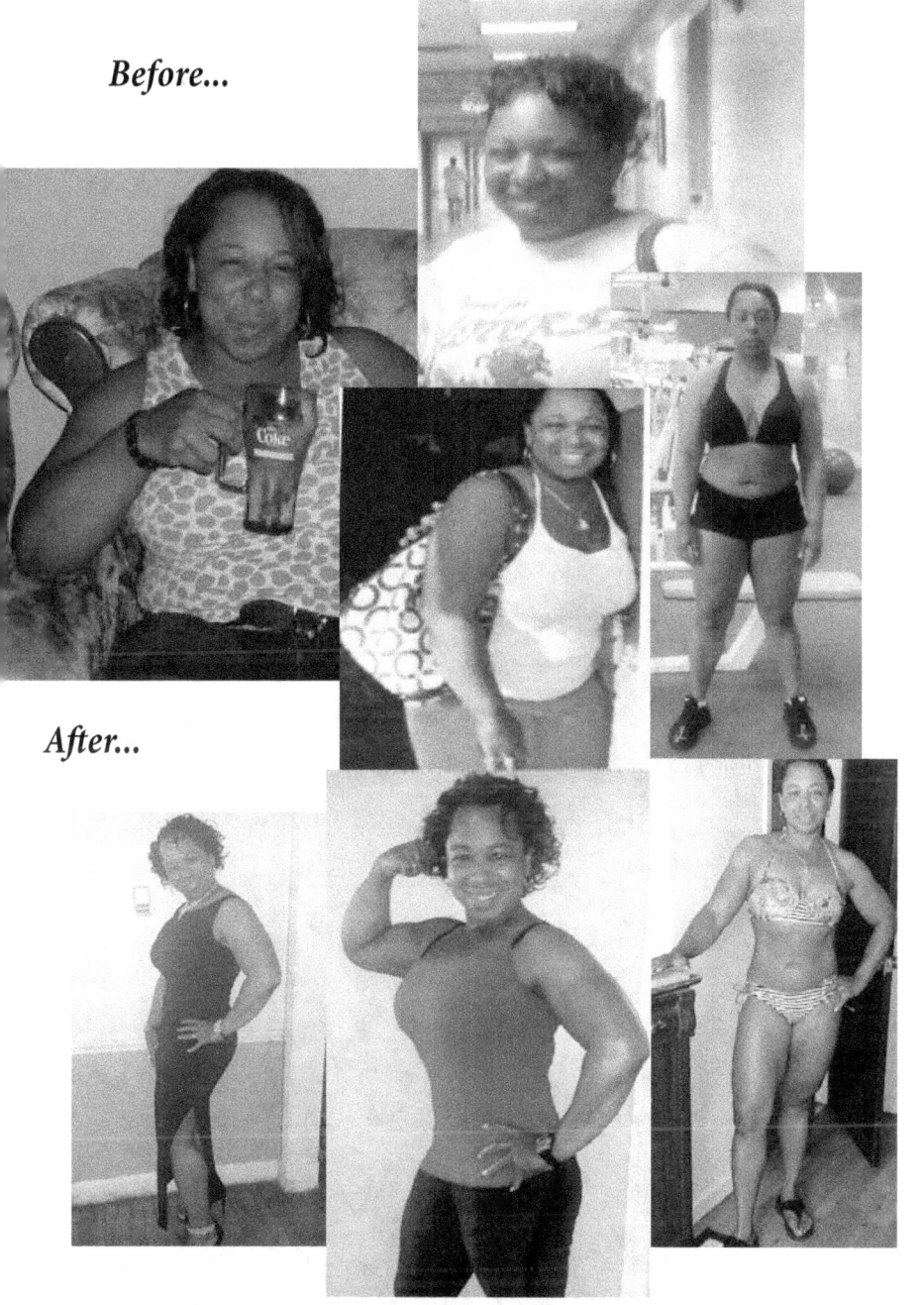

Nick

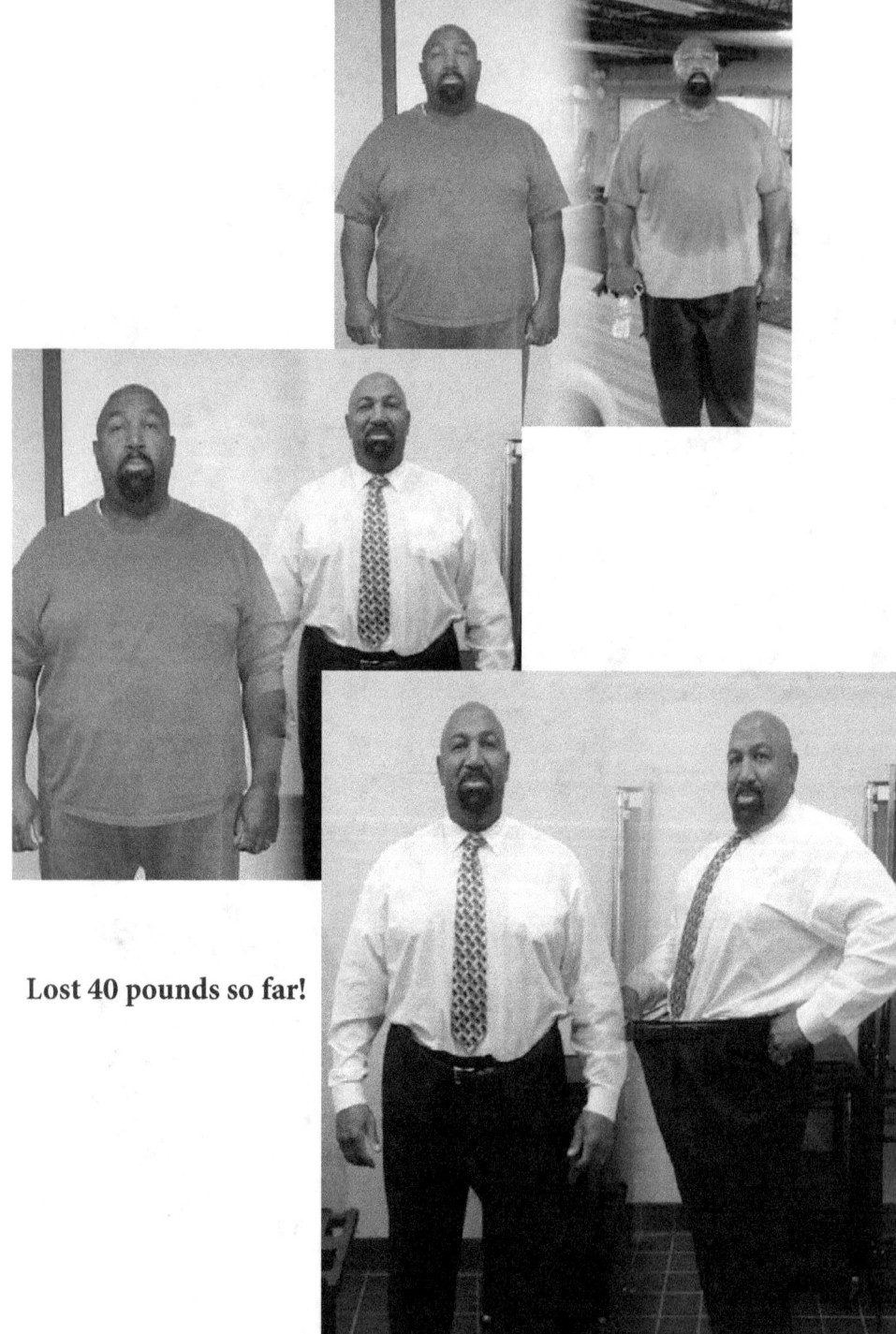

Lost 40 pounds so far!

Michele

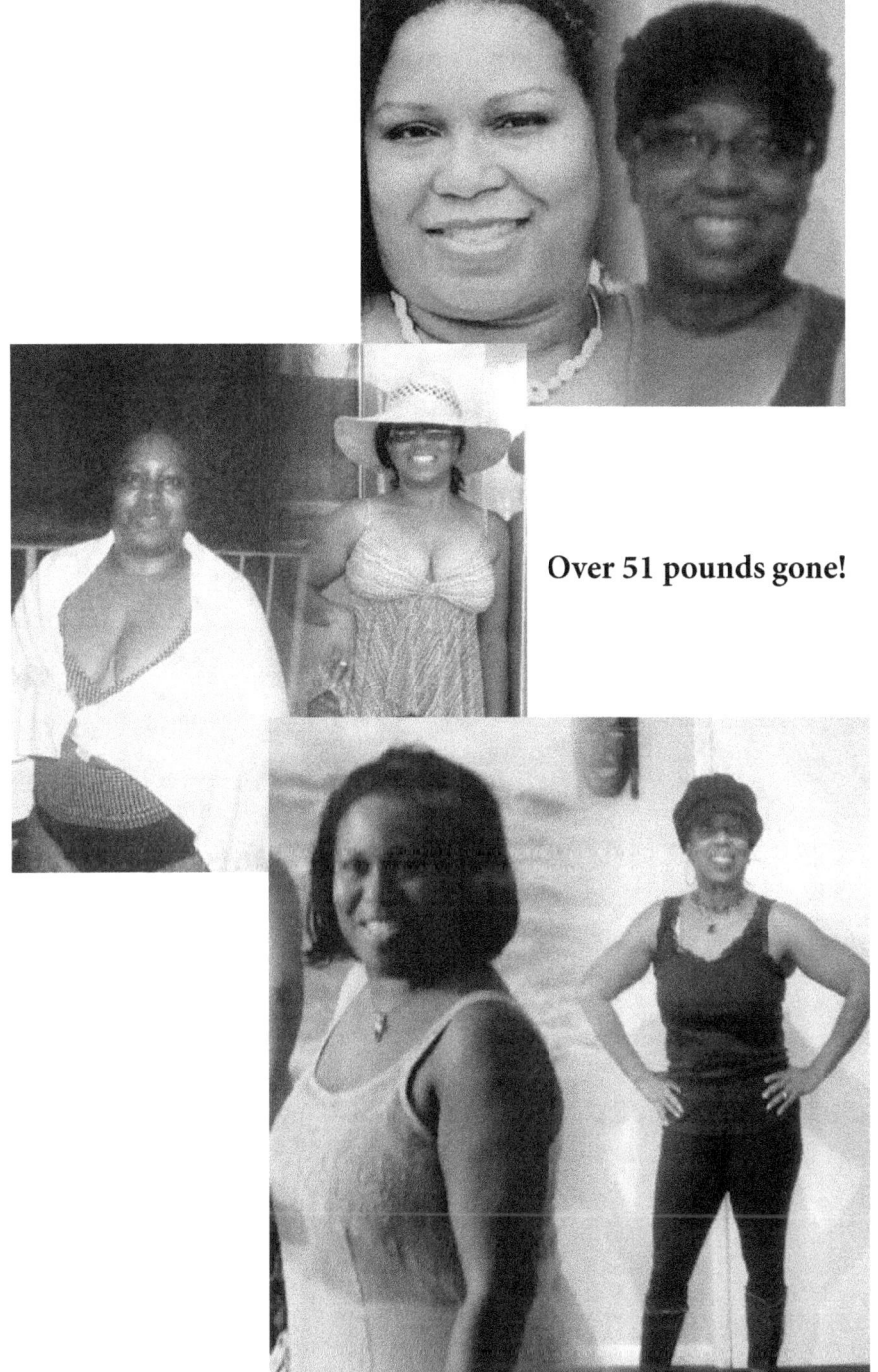

Over 51 pounds gone!

References

References

Dr. Josh Axe, DNM, DC, CNS, certified Doctor of Natural Medicine, Doctor of Chiropractic and Clinical Nutrition9, DHEA

"Testosterone and Androgens in Women," Monash University (medicine, nursing and health science), October 2010

"What is Menopause?" National Institute on Aging, National Institutes of Health U.S. Department of Health and Human Services, Pub. December 2013

"Menopause & Heart Disease," American Heart Association, July 2015

"Protein Power," Dr. Michael R. Eades and Mary Dan Eades MD, February 1996

"Exercise & Menstruation: Training with your cycle (Female Phase Training)," blog, Dr. Jade Teta, May 24, 2013

"Skeletal muscle metabolism is a major determinant of resting energy expenditure. (ref muscle-metabolism)," F. Zurlo, K. Larson, C. Bogardus, and E. Ravussin, Journal List, J Clin Invest, v.86(5); 1990 Nov, PMC296885

"Prevalence of Obesity Among Adults and Youth: United States, 2011–2014," National Center for Health Statistics, Cynthia L. Ogden, Ph.D.; Margaret D. Carroll, M.S.P.H.; Cheryl D. Fryar, M.S.P.H.; and Katherine M. Flegal, Ph.D., https://www.census.gov/population

"Metabolic obesity: the paradox between visceral and subcutaneous fat," Joslin Diabetes Center, Harvard Medical School, Boston, MA 02215, USA, osama.hamdy@joslin.harvard.edu

"Abdominal Obesity and Your Health," Harvard Medical School, Harvard Health Publication, September 2005

"Red wine and resveratrol good for your heart," The Mayo Clinc, http://www.mayoclinic.org/diseases-conditions/heart-disease/in-depth/red-wine/art-20048281

"Each Organ Has a Unique Metabolic Profile," NCBA, Brain Sugar; 2002, W. H. Freeman and Company.Bookshelf ID: NBK22436

"Burn the Fat, Feed the Muscle," Tom Venuto, December 2013

"FDA Cuts trans fats in processed foods," https://www.fda.gov/ForConsumers/ConsumerUpdates/ucm372915.htm

"World Health Organization Europe leads the world in eliminating trans fats," Copenhagen, 18 September 2014, http://www.euro.who.int/en/media-centre/sections/press-releases/2014/europe-leads-the-world-in-eliminating-trans-fats

"Prescription for Nutrional Healing," Susan A. Balch CNC, 3rd Addition, 2000

"EPA chief refuses to ban pesticide," http://www.huffingtonpost.com/entry/scott-pruitt-pesticide-chlorpyrifos_us_58dd331de4b0e6ac7092fbd8

"The water in you," H.H. Mitchell, Journal of Biological Chemistry, 158, https://water.usgs.gov/edu/propertyyou.html

"Coffee caffeine content," https://ndb.nal.usda.gov/ndb/foods/show/4277

"Six reasons to drink coffee before your workout," http://fitness.mercola.com/sites/fitness/archive/2014/07/11/6-coffee-pre-workout-benefits.aspx

"Avoid the Trans Fat Trap," http://www.shape.com/blogs/weight-loss-coach/avoid-trans-fat-trap

"How much sodium will I eat per day," https://sodiumbreakup.heart.org/how_much_sodium_should_i_eat?utm_source=SRI&utm_medium=HeartOrg&utm_term=Website&utm_content=SodiumAndSalt&utm_campaign=SodiumBreakup

"What's the difference between sea salt and table salt?" http://www.mayoclinic.org/healthy-lifestyle/nutrition-and-healthy-eating/expert-answers/sea-salt/faq-20058512

"Carbs, Not Fats, Boost Half-Marathon Race Performance, Study Finds," http://www.the-aps.org/mm/hp/Audiences/Public-Press/2015-69.html

"Quanity and Quality of Exercise," ACSM, http://www.acsm.org/about-acsm/media-room/news-releases/2011/08/01/acsm-issues-new-recommendations-on-quantity-and-quality-of-exercise

"Too much cardio can cause a 7 fold surge of heart problems," http://fitness.mercola.com/sites/fitness/archive/2012/06/01/long-cardio-workout-dangers.aspx

"The swim suit diet," Metabolic Effect, Dr. Jade Teta, 2016

"Green tea research," International journey of Obesity, July 14, 2009,
http://www.umm.edu/health/medical/altmed/herb/green-tea

"Spot reduction," http://ajsportscentre.com.au/fitness-myths-ignore/

"Bureau of Labor Statistics, Fitness Trainers," December 17, 2015,
 https://www.bls.gov/ooh/personal-care-and-service/fitness-trainers-and-in-
structors.htm#tab-6

"Everything you need to know about intermittent fasting,"

How to be

Fit

Fabulous

Fortified

& *free*

www.ingramcontent.com/pod-product-compliance
Lightning Source LLC
Chambersburg PA
CBHW071201280526
45787CB00002B/560